Decision Maki
Paramedic Practice

Andy Collen

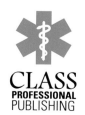

CLASS
PROFESSIONAL
PUBLISHING

This edition first published 2017
Reprinted in 2018, 2019 with corrections, 2020

The publishers and author welcome feedback from readers of this book.

Class Professional Publishing
The Exchange, Express Park, Bristol Road, Bridgwater TA6 4RR
Email: info@class.co.uk
www.classprofessional.co.uk

Class Professional Publishing is an imprint of Class Publishing Ltd

A CIP catalogue record for this book is available from the British Library

Paperback ISBN: 978-1859596418
eBook ISBN: 978-1859596425

Cover design by Hybert Design Limited, UK

Designed and typeset by RefineCatch Limited, www.refinecatch.com

Printed in the UK by Hobbs the Printers Ltd, Totton, Hampshire, UK

For my wife Debbie, and my boys, Toby & Will.
Three of the best decisions I have made.

About the Author

Andy Collen is a Consultant Paramedic at South East Coast Ambulance Service (SECAmb) and has worked as a Safety Investigator for the Healthcare Safety Investigation Branch. He is also the Medicines and Prescribing Project Lead for the College of Paramedics, working with NHS England and other Allied Health Professional (AHP) bodies on the proposal to extend non-medical prescribing, including the work to introduce independent prescribing for advanced paramedics. He has been in the NHS since 1989, and progressed through a traditional ambulance service career, qualifying as a paramedic in 2000. After qualifying as a specialist paramedic in 2006, he left the ambulance service to practise in a walk-in centre in order to develop his skills. He returned to the ambulance service full time in 2009 to lead the specialist paramedic programmes and to work on improving professional careers and clinical leadership. He completed a MSc in 2013 and was appointed to his consultant post in 2015.

Andy sits on the Ambulance Lead Paramedic Group and the National Ambulance Urgent and Emergency Care Group. He previously contributed to the *JRCALC Guidelines* and the UK edition of *Emergency Care in the Streets*. He undertakes sessional lectures on decision making at universities in the South East region and has presented extensively on the prescribing project across the UK.

When not working in a professional capacity, Andy is a drummer and music fan. Most importantly, he enjoys spending time with his family.

Contents

Contents

Foreword *by Professor Andy Newton, Past Chair, College of Paramedics*

The time is right for this book, marking as it does one of the greatest and most far reaching changes that paramedics face today, specifically the need for ever more complex decision making. This is particularly true in regard to the changing epidemiologic context of our time, characterised by increasing patient complexity, itself driven by different patterns of demography. Although not always fully recognised by policy makers, senior NHS managers and indeed authors of paramedic textbooks, these factors are ever more tangible and require a response in the form of an evolution of the paramedic role, from a first contact provider to one who can assess patient need in a range of circumstances and, where possible, treat and discharge if appropriate.

To address these challenges, Andy Collen has built a text which offers not only a brief introduction to these changes, but also subsequently reinforces the professional issues and responsibilities which underpin safe clinical practice every bit as much as knowledge of anatomy and physiology do. Many current paramedic degree programmes do of course provide some grounding in areas such as ethics, reflective practice and the regulatory context of practice, although vocational programmes have often skirted around these topics. It is therefore apposite that effort is expended revisiting, amplifying and considering in more detail these factors, thereby making for more inclusive and well-rounded text than might otherwise be the case.

By designing his book in this way, Andy Collen ensures that the reader is well prepared for the next phase of discussion: developing critical reasoning and decision making. These are again increasingly essential aspects of practice that, while now firmly embedded in the paramedic undergraduate programme, can hardly be over-emphasised. Equally, the importance of team working as a precursor to ensuring good clinical practice is considered with reference to human factors. Other industries that operate in a safety critical environment, such as aviation, the military, policing and fire services, have had the benefit of additional preparation in this area for many years. It is therefore an extremely positive development that these areas are integrated into paramedic practice in this publication.

This book has many strengths and is certainly a timely addition to the range of textbooks available for paramedics. It also reflects the continued need to highlight the facets of clinical decision making and hone these skills to ensure that paramedic practice remains entirely reflective of emerging patient need. Personally, I particularly liked the case studies and felt that they provided precisely the type of substrate that helped to effectively illustrate the material in general. Given the ever more exciting work that paramedics undertake in today's high-pressure environment, where there is less and less room for tolerance of errors, this book provides a valuable contribution that will no doubt appeal to paramedics everywhere.

1 Paramedic Practice: The Changing Patient Profile in Urgent, Emergency and Critical Care

Chapter Objectives

This chapter will cover:

- The development of the paramedic;
- The evolving role of paramedics and changing practice settings;
- Patient **demography** and **epidemiology**;
- Professional conduct and standards;
- The paramedic's role as an Allied Health Professional.

Introduction: The Development of the Paramedic

The term 'paramedic' emerged in the UK from the well-established title used in North America. It was adopted for early schemes in Brighton and Bristol which, prior to the formal adoption of the term, went on to drive the 'extended care' ambulance service roles developed in the mid-1980s. A standard paramedic curriculum became established in the early 1990s. By 2000, paramedics were able to register with the Council for Professions Supplementary to Medicine (CPSM), which went on to become the Healthcare Professions Council (HPC) and more recently the Health and Care Professions Council (**HCPC**). This registration, initially voluntary, became compulsory in 2003, which is the year the HPC published its first edition of the *Standards of Proficiency for Paramedics*.

In the context of decision making, the paramedic needed to develop into a profession whose members were truly professional and were responsible for their actions through regulation. This change occurred in the early 2000s, saw paramedics considered 'broadly autonomous', and implied significant responsibility to intervene in highly complex clinical scenarios, albeit with little or no supervision or support. The professionalising of what was previously a largely vocational role, created by **rote learning** and training rather than higher education, was extremely rapid. In many ways the profession is still in transition. The dawning of the era of paramedic regulation, and the events of the following decade, coincided with changes to many aspects of paramedic practice – not least the increasing diversity of paramedic practice settings. The details of the changing and emerging patient profiles are covered later in this chapter, but the main changes affecting paramedics and the services they work for are due to the requirement to provide care for an increasingly ageing population. Many of these older people, who often have one or more long-term health conditions, are living alone and independently in the community, and this inevitably impacts on demand for care. Linked to this, the illnesses and injuries traditionally associated with paramedic practice, such as vehicle trauma, are declining due to changes to car design and improved driver and passenger safety measures (such as crumple zones and airbags). This era has also seen more focus on prevention, and a shift in public attitude towards a reduction in drink driving, and greater use of seatbelts. In 1980 there were 5,953 deaths on the roads in the UK; this fell to 1,713 in 2013 (DoT, 2014). While trauma can still be complex, the decision to admit patients to hospital with long bone fractures, head and internal injuries, rarely needed much deliberation as patients' ongoing care for these conditions is largely pre-determined and could only be provided in secondary care. While that is still true now, the changing proportions of patients not needing secondary care has grown exponentially.

The combined effect of these changes meant that paramedics began to be required to make more complex decisions for a larger number of patients with a growing range of needs. While the critical care role has always existed, and will continue to develop, fewer cases can now be described as high **acuity**/low complexity and more as low acuity/high complexity (see Figure 1.1).

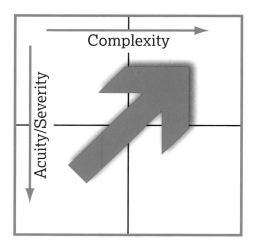

Figure 1.1: *The shift of patient presentations seen by paramedics*

One the most important developments for the paramedic profession was the establishment of the professional body (College of Paramedics, 2017). Professional bodies are common to all registered healthcare professions and are vital in representing the interests of their membership. The College of Paramedics is responsible for the development of curricula documents, career guidance and competency frameworks. It also provides membership services such as medical indemnity insurance and malpractice cover, as well as organising annual national conferences and regional events. The College of Paramedics also works closely with

Health Education England and the higher education institutes to ensure that the paramedic profession remains fit for purpose, and undergraduate and postgraduate courses are of sufficient quality.

It is only through the development of the profession that the rapid pace of change has been possible. While this has had significant benefit for patients, the healthcare system, and the paramedics themselves, it must be remembered that with these developments comes more responsibility. Increasingly, paramedics are required to make more and more complex decisions.

HCPC Standards

The Health and Care Professions Council standards are central to professional practice and the following points are taken from their standards of conduct, performance and ethics. These points underpin much of what is discussed in the rest of this chapter. They remind the paramedic of aspects to practice which are vitally important such as communication skills, personal conduct and acting in the patient's best interests. Decision making requires the paramedic to ensure they are fully informed, and to actively seek the amount of information required to make a decision. While most information is easily accessible (it can be seen, read, heard, smelled etc.), other factors are either inaccessible (and require further enquiry or examination) or hidden in plain sight (but you may not know what to look for). Make sure you are aware of the standards required in practice, and use them to help you with your developing decision-making skills.

Registrants must:

- promote and protect the interests of service users and carers;
- communicate appropriately and effectively;
- work within the limits of their knowledge and skills;
- delegate appropriately;
- respect confidentiality;
- manage risk;
- report concerns about safety;
- be open when things go wrong;
- be honest and trustworthy; and
- keep records of their work.

(HCPC, 2016)

The Evolving Role of Paramedics and Changing Practice Settings

The paramedic role is evolving rapidly with greater opportunity to practise across a range of settings, spanning the career framework, and with far more mobility than previously experienced by paramedics. Traditional roles for paramedics rarely extended beyond employment in an ambulance trust, either in clinical roles or as managers or trainers. This confinement restricted the potential for paramedics to be seen in the wider health economies for many years. Arguably, the most significant change to paramedic practice came with the publication of *Taking Healthcare to the Patient* (DH, 2005); this document describes a broadening of roles for paramedics, focusing on providing healthcare rather than simply transport as well as laying the foundations for a diversification of practice settings. At the same time, early pilots of what we now recognise as specialist and advanced practice roles were being developed, allowing paramedics to return to, or undertake for the first time, higher education study in more depth on many essential practical and theoretical concepts. Paramedics emerged initially from a role which looked only at signs and symptoms ahead of taking the patient to the hospital, and decision making may have extended only as far as which hospital was closest.

This leap forward, which has now developed into a more consistent professional career framework, needed to be underpinned by better education and training for those joining the profession. This has become essential and is supported by a range of evidence including most importantly the *Paramedic Evidence Based Education Project* (Lovegrove and Davis, 2013). This advocates strongly for the change to undergraduate education, moving to all paramedics registering for the first time needing a Bachelor's Degree. These changes have all contributed to paramedics' potential being recognised more widely. In 2011, the second edition of *Taking Healthcare to the Patient* (AACE, 2011) made suggestions including a proposal to introduce independent prescribing, supporting a consultation published in 2010. The basis for the proposal for independent prescribing is that the paramedic in an advanced practice role is suitably equipped to make excellent decisions, and can diagnose and treat patients in a range of settings. At the time of writing, in 2017, independent prescribing is still to become a reality. However, the proposal was discussed by the Commission on Human Medicines in late 2015, and again in 2016, bringing it a step closer. If passed eventually, it will provide safer and more timely access to medicines for those patients who are being treated by paramedics.

Paramedics are no longer synonymous with ambulances or ambulance services, which is good news for patients and the profession. The support given to the paramedic professional in recent years, such as in the *Urgent and Emergency Care Review* produced by Professor Sir Bruce Keogh, Medical Director for NHS England, has given paramedics roles in a much wider range of practice settings (NHS England, 2013). Paramedics now work in GP practices, emergency departments, out of hours services, community services, aeromedical services, motorsport medicine, military healthcare, and expedition medicine, as well as the more traditional roles in ambulance services and helicopter emergency medical services (**HEMS**). The career opportunities for those entering the profession are rich and diverse, and the breadth of settings often include much more inter-professional and multi-professional working, seeing teams formed from other **Allied Health Professionals** (AHPs), nurses and doctors, as well as mental health professionals, social care professions and staff from other agencies. Paramedics do not just work alongside the police and fire brigade anymore, and are positioned firmly as Allied Health Professionals.

To be trusted as a healthcare professional, it is vital for the paramedic to be seen as a decision maker in order to represent him- or herself consistently according to their core professional identity. The opportunities which exist must be approached as an opportunity to focus on ensuring patients have the best access to high-quality care from a range of skilled healthcare professionals, each with their own unique skills and abilities, coming together to define the nature of multi-professionalism. The risk of making healthcare professions generic may dilute the unique core skills of paramedics, as well as those of the other AHPs and nurses. All these professions run the risk of being viewed as interchangeable because of the apparent similarity of intent when providing care. In reality though, this may damage the patient/carer relationship. Paramedics who move up the Career Framework (College of Paramedics, 2015) and into diverse practice settings remain paramedics and must uphold the standards published by their professional regulator, the Health and Care Professions Council. Registrants cannot abdicate their professional title – most importantly they cannot adopt another role title that creates a misrepresentation during the care encounter. We should be proud of our profession and ensure that we promote it – celebrating the time when we approach a patient and introduce ourselves as a paramedic.

The ever-growing range of practice settings is raising the profile of paramedics and placing them within care teams which previously were occupied by one profession alone. The College of Paramedics Career Framework (2015), and its accompanying curriculum guidance, demonstrates the diversity of paramedic practice (see Figure 1.2). Whether you are a graduate starting your first job with an ambulance trust, or an advanced paramedic working in a multi-professional environment, the two axes which describe the professional demonstrate the advances paramedics have made since their inception in the early 1980s – as clinicians, practitioners, critical thinkers, educators, researchers and, most importantly, decision makers.

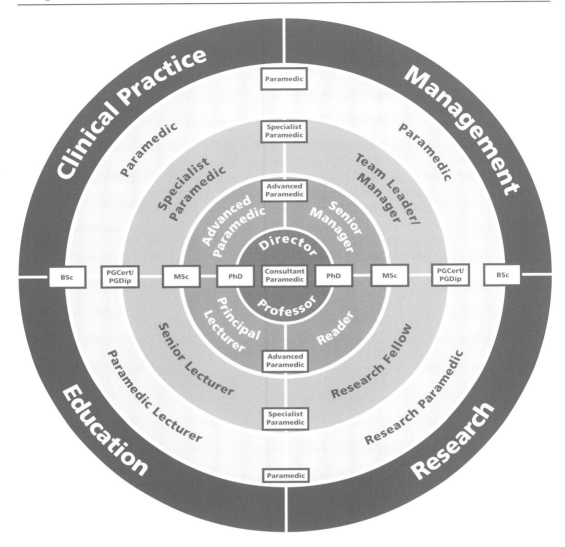

Figure 1.2: *College of Paramedics' Career Framework (2015)*

Patient Demography and Epidemiology

In real terms, there are twice the number of 999 calls to ambulance services each year compared to a decade ago (NHS Digital, 2014). Paramedics are seeing more and more patients in other practice settings outside the traditional ambulance service environment, such as GP practices, urgent care centres and emergency departments. Patients with long-term health conditions, such as COPD (chronic obstructive pulmonary disease), diabetes, Parkinson's disease etc., make up around 50% of all appointments in primary care each year and account for 70% of all inpatient bed days (Kings Fund, 2016). This underpins the importance of good decision making when providing care for these patients, not only in relation to the direct care for the individual patient, but in the context of the economic impact of long-term healthcare on society. Patients with long-term health problems pose a greater challenge for the decision maker as their condition may present more complex information and considerations. For example, patients with COPD may have lower oxygen saturation, and this must be taken into account when dealing with an acute problem.

'In England, more than 15 million people have a long-term condition – a health problem that can't be cured but can be controlled by medication or other therapies. This figure is set to increase over the next 10 years, particularly those people with 3 or more conditions at once. Examples of long-term conditions include high blood pressure, depression, dementia and arthritis.'

(DH, 2015)

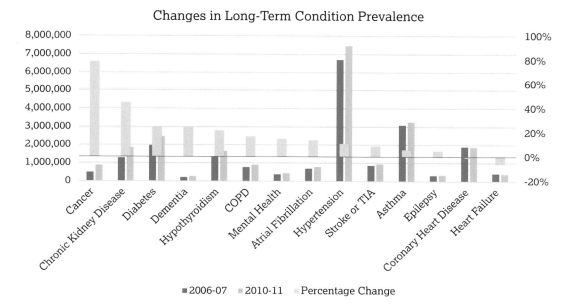

Figure 1.3: *Changes in Long-Term Condition Prevalence*

Across the whole of health and social care, £7 out of every £10 is spent on care for patients with long-term healthcare needs. The problem is compounded as care becomes more complex from the perspective of **multi-morbidity** with around 30% of the population having one or more long-term health conditions (DH, 2012). The population is getting older, adding further challenges associated with the normal changes seen in ageing and how these can impact on the prevalence and management of long-term healthcare (see Figure 1.3) – particularly when considered in the context of promoting independent living in the community.

Patients with long-term health conditions are increasing in numbers and account for significant resource use across health and social care. For paramedics, contact with these patients often occurs at times of crisis and therefore these encounters are complex. Decision making in relation to the **comorbid** patient suffering an acute-on-chronic presentation, which may also potentially involve considerations relating to advanced decisions and end of life care, can lead to the risk of avoidable hospital admission and failure to meet care goals. Health policy is moving towards care closer to home (NHS England, 2013) and therefore paramedics must consider how to make the best decision for patients across the spectrum of age and disease. Later chapters look at the dilemmas and conundrums faced in practice, and discuss scenarios relating to patients with long-term healthcare needs.

By way of summary, people with long-term conditions account for:

- 50% of all GP appointments;
- 64% of outpatient appointments;
- 70% of all inpatient bed days;
- In total around 70% of the total health and care spend in England (£7 out of every £10);

This means that 30% of the population account for 70% of the spend.

(DH, 2012, p.3)

People with long-term conditions consistently say:

- They want to be involved in decisions about their care – they want to be listened to;
- They want access to information to help them make those decisions;
- They want support to understand their condition and confidence to manage – support to self-care;
- They want joined up, seamless services;
- They want proactive care;
- They do not want to be in hospital unless it is absolutely necessary and then only as part of a planned approach;
- They want to be treated as a whole person and for the NHS to act as one team.

(DH, 2012, p.3)

Patients with long-term healthcare problems are a growing cohort and are usually complex. Improving the approach to decision making for this group of patients is vital for paramedics if they are to contribute effectively to the health of the nation and to support healthcare policy in action – most importantly ensuring that patients' voices are heard and their wishes met. Long-term disease prevalence and multi-morbidity cannot however be seen in isolation; there are two more important aspects to care – ageing and deprivation – which impact on decision making and often exist alongside long-term healthcare problems as a triad.

The UK population is getting older (see Figure 1.4) and the prevalence of multi-morbidity increases with age, and in the presence of deprivation. The population of the UK is expected to increase by around 3% between 2015 and 2020 and, within this general rise, the number of people aged 65 and over will increase by 1.1 million, an equivalent of 12%. Within this period the number of people aged over 85 will increase by 300,000, and there will be 7,000 more people reaching their century. In the early 1990s it was truly rare for a paramedic to attend a patient aged 100 or over, whereas now it is far less unusual and only noteworthy where 100 has been exceeded by several years.

Ageing in itself is not a disease, but the anatomical, physiological and psychological changes experienced in ageing are important to underlying health. Older patients are more prone to illness, often associated with age and frailty. This results in patients living independently or in supported living in the community, doing so with increased risks to their health, secondary to their age. For instance, an older patient with diminished bone density and **polypharmacy** is at far higher risk of falling and suffering a fracture. Patients who have already suffered a fracture over the age of 65 are far more likely to suffer another 'fragility fracture' as a result of subsequent falls. The decision making for this group of patients, therefore, is increasingly complex – considering carefully the risk/benefit balance of promoting independent living versus admission to hospital in the face of increased risk of an injurious fall. This can only be done in the presence of good decision making which ensures the patient is paramount, and their wishes are considered in the context of the information they need to make an informed decision about their own healthcare.

While epidemiology and demography are the main areas of analysis most commonly seen in health data, at a practical level clinicians need to consider the concept of deprivation in the context of the wider background information available. Deprivation is in essence the lack of basic means to live at a level associated with good health and wellbeing:

> '... a situation in which you do not have things or conditions that are usually considered necessary for a pleasant life.'
>
> (Cambridge Dictionary, 2017)

Deprivation impacts on individual patients' health and wellbeing, and life expectancy. Also, the instances of long-term ill health increase where deprivation is seen. Many paramedics will be familiar with its symptoms. It is often seen in clusters, and when these are linked by geography this can give the impression that everyone in that area is deprived, but the following statement demonstrates that this is not true:

> 'It is important to note that these statistics are a measure of relative deprivation, not affluence, and to recognise that not every person in a highly-deprived area will themselves be deprived. Likewise, there will be some deprived people living in the least deprived areas.'
>
> (DCLG, 2015)

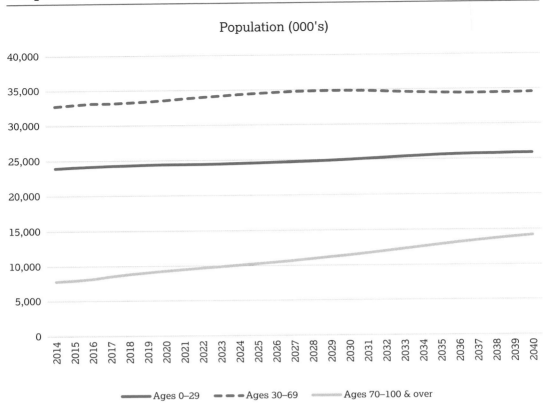

Figure 1.4: *The changing shape of the UK population (information taken from the ONS, 2015)*

For the decision maker, deprivation must be considered in the context of the diagnostic and treatment process. For instance, the instances of undiagnosed long-term disease are more prevalent in areas of deprivation which means that it is in these areas that you are more likely to see patients with COPD that has not been formally diagnosed or managed. This is also reflected in life expectancy, with significant differences in average lifespans in Wokingham and Manchester, or Richmond and Tower Hamlets (DCLG, 2015).

Decision making has many cues and places from which better formed ideas can be tested. Consideration must be given to all the factors that assist with making a better decision. Working in certain areas, or working with certain defined groups (such as by age or deprivation), consideration can be given to increasing the context of care in these settings, and while this is not the main influence in making a decision, it helps with the richness of the analysis and therefore the quality of the result for the patient.

Professional Conduct and Standards

'Professionalism' can sometimes be a vague and somewhat nebulous term, often implied rather than bestowed, and with a sense that one can unconditionally adopt professionalism by dint of a qualification. While this may not be consistent with the emerging evidence, one could be forgiven for not fully appreciating what professionalism is. *The Oxford English Dictionary* (2013) has a comprehensive entry relating to the words 'professional' and 'professionalism' and these include:

- *'Senses relating to or derived from (the conduct of) a profession or occupation.'*

- *'Of a person or persons: that engages in a specified occupation or activity for money or as a means of earning a living, rather than as a pastime. Contrasted with amateur.'*

- *'Relating to, connected with, or befitting a (particular) profession or calling; preliminary or necessary to the practice of a profession.'*

- *'Engaged in a profession, esp. one requiring special skill or training; belonging to the professional classes.'*

- *'That has or displays the skill, knowledge, experience, standards, or expertise of a professional; competent, efficient.'*

- *'That has knowledge of the theoretical or scientific parts of a trade or occupation, as distinct from its practical or mechanical aspects; that raises a trade to a learned profession.'*

(OED, 2013)

Being a member of a profession may not link to professionalism in all cases, but in healthcare, the values and behaviours which ensure that patients are treated effectively, safely and with dignity are vital to the point where professionalism exists as a feature alongside competent technical skill. Paramedics are, by definition, healthcare professionals and are registered and regulated accordingly. However, professionalism is achieved with a far more objective range of values, in many ways distinct from competency. For example, and in the context of decision making, unprofessional behaviour may be seen where a patient for whom admission to the emergency department is not indicated is taken there by a paramedic who wants a cup of tea (which they know they can get there). In **biomedical ethics**, the patient must never be the *means to an end* – they must only ever be *the end* in itself – to paraphrase Immanuel Kant (1724–1804). This means that the good of the patient must be considered above other considerations; the patient should never be used as a means of achieving another goal – such as by leveraging the system to visit the place the paramedic wants to be (to get a cup of tea) rather than where the patient needs to be. Using the patient as a lever to visit the local hospital is unprofessional, and the decision making which leads to this is flawed.

We will explore throughout this book how the process of decision making is linked to other considerations, and professionalism is assumed throughout rather than being added as a constant reminder. It is important therefore to reflect on professionalism as a concept. This will promote optimal 'purity' in decision making, free from the extrinsic factors and stressors which may result in deviation from the focus essential to patient/carer relationship. Basing practice on high professional standards in many ways makes decision making easier. It is an exercise that can be used to enhance professional fitness and therefore confidence and competence in practice.

So, how is professionalism defined and understood? Using the findings from the Consensus towards Understanding and Sustaining Professionalism in Paramedic Practice study (Gallagher et al., 2016), we can see how the profession defines professionalism for itself, both from among practising clinicians and those invited to contribute to the Delphi Study which formed part of the research study. The key findings suggest that paramedic professionalism has four components:

- The conduct and character of paramedics;
- The role of regulation;
- Professional education;
- The values that paramedics profess.

The professionalism enablers identified by this project revealed a good deal of consensus regarding participants' views of broader factors that impact on professionalism. These are the role of regulation, regulators' codes and standards, professional education and the responses of the general public. There were suggestions also that other professions, such as GPs, do not always give paramedics the respect they deserve. The data also highlights the view that responsibility for paramedic professionalism goes beyond individuals, with organisations having a key role in providing support. The role of employers in promoting and enacting professional values was also highlighted as an important professionalism enabler.

There is further discussion in Chapter 6 on professional issues, including the responsibilities associated with being a registered healthcare professional.

The Paramedic's Role as an Allied Health Professional

Paramedics are Allied Health Professionals (AHPs) alongside other professions such as physiotherapists, dietitians, radiographers, speech and language therapists, orthoptists, podiatrists, occupational therapists, prosthetists/orthotists, drama therapists, art therapists, and music therapists. The term Allied Health Professional (AHP) is an extremely important aspect of practice for paramedics. There are 130,000 AHPs registered in the UK, of which only around 20,000 are paramedics. The 12 AHPs are represented by the Allied Health Professions Federation which acts on behalf the individual professions to provide collective leadership on issues common to all AHPs (AHPF, 2016).

Paramedics are recognised as central to the delivery of high-quality healthcare in the community, and this increasing recognition and responsibility means that each paramedic must be able to do the very best for their patients. This means making decisions every day of their working lives. Being part of the wider family of Allied Health Professionals is important for paramedics. It also promotes multi-professional and inter-professional working, which has clear benefits for patients.

Paramedics are unique in comparison to other AHPs as their area of practice is generalised and occupying a wide breadth of practice. In reality, paramedics are focused on patients with a well-defined range of conditions, which are linked by their onset or severity. Most other AHPs, in contrast, provide care in a more planned way. Paramedics should understand their role as an AHP and be aware of the roles of the other AHPs as there are always opportunities to refer to other professions. While it is less likely a paramedic will refer patients to art therapists or drama therapists, they will interact with physiotherapists, occupational therapists, dietitians and radiographers far more often. It is important, therefore, to understand what all these professions can offer your patients. Developing this understanding will also enhance your professional knowledge.

Just as regulation with the HCPC is important for paramedics as professionals, so too is membership of the professional body, the College of Paramedics. Paramedics should also have an awareness of themselves as members of an Allied Health Profession, as this is equally important for sharing best practice. Embracing the common values of AHPs can only enhance their knowledge and effectiveness in practice. In addition, the Allied Health Professions Federation exists to represent the interests of AHPs in areas common to their members. You can find out more about the AHPF at www.ahpf.org.uk.

Conclusion

Paramedic practice is no longer as simple as putting someone on a stretcher and driving them to hospital. Moreover, paramedics are not just working in the ambulance setting and are working across a range of multi-professional practice settings, such as primary care, emergency departments, military, offshore, remote medicine, and private practice. Ambulance services provide very basic professional leadership, and often promote a top-down approach to professional responsibility. In reality, and in response to our evolving profession, paramedics need to look across other professions and sectors in order to understand fully the requirements of professional practice. Decision making must be one of the cornerstones of professional practice as it underpins and promotes safety during clinical encounters – regardless of the practice setting. Without objective decision making, any imbalance between confidence and competence can be dangerous; therefore, professional responsibility and **autonomy** should be considered carefully in the context of self-awareness and the risks associated with biased thinking.

Patients are changing too. They are more informed about their health and have greater expectations about the healthcare they receive. Patient-centred care means that all healthcare professionals must make the correct decisions about each individual patient's care, and these decisions must be reached on the basis that the patient is paramount. As professional practice has developed and become more complex, healthcare professionals must become better at decision making in order to create the best outcome for patients.

The next chapter introduces some of the issues and considerations which run alongside clinical practice. While these may not be directly associated with decision making, they do provide an important context for professional practice, and therefore influence everything we do for our patients.

Reflective Exercises

- Consider your own role in clinical practice and reflect on your own professional development, taking into account the ageing population and the increasingly complex patients for whom paramedics provide care.

- What do professional and regulatory standards mean to you? Consider the key documents published by the HCPC at this stage of your development in relation to making decisions. (You may want to repeat this reflective exercise after reading Chapter 6.)

- What does it mean to be an Allied Health Professional? In relation to decision making, what similarities and differences are there between professions?

2 Professional Issues

Chapter Objectives

This chapter will cover:

- Professional regulation and standards;
- Professional identity;
- Biomedical ethics;
- Patient-centred care;
- Confidentiality;
- Competence and confidence in practice;
- Professional insight.

Introduction

In order to make decisions for, and with, your patients, it is important to fully understand the constellation of other factors and considerations which guide and regulate professional practice. Many of the aspects discussed in this chapter are not directly related to decision making theory, but are important concepts to consider and reflect upon as intrinsic aspects of your day-to-day clinical practice. The care you provide is done so, directly or indirectly, in line with published standards, ethical considerations, laws and legislation, best practice guidance, and patient-focused principles. Personal integrity plays a significant role in professional practice, and displaying insight into your practice helps to weave together your knowledge, skills and competencies into a **holistic acumen** upon which good decisions can be built.

Professional clinical practice involves a significant amount of personal sacrifice, study, long hours, bearing witness to traumatic events and, most importantly, being registered with a regulating body. This is balanced against the privilege of being invited into patients' lives at their time of need; striving to save their life or minimising the impact of the disease that has befallen them. The concepts of harm and error are discussed throughout this book, and this chapter covers many of the aspects of professional practice which can overwhelm paramedics when thinking about consequence.

To be an effective clinician, it is vital to promote confidence in your practice. There are plenty of opportunities to create anxiety – particularly associated with making complex decisions, and that often insidious threat (perceived or actual) of consequences when things go wrong. We will explore some of these factors in the context of decision making and reflecting how to further understand and minimise risk, particularly relating to professional considerations. It is extremely rare for errors to be made intentionally – no one comes to work to do a bad job. Where problems arise, judgements are made more commonly in the context of reasonable actions and opportunities to learn. The NHS promotes a **learning culture**, and this is increasingly being balanced against the need to apply a just approach to errors. Being prepared, competent, and able to make defensible decisions – rather than practising defensively – is a way of ensuring your clinical practice is safe and rewarding.

There are a range of issues involving decision making, and these include concepts such as patient-centred care, confidentiality, impartiality, biomedical ethics and reflection. This chapter will link these areas of learning, and the concepts presented, in the context of these considerations. This chapter is intended to add colour to your emerging and developing decision-making acumen, ensuring that one avoids becoming a 'decision making robot', and retains the safe holistic approach to care that patients deserve, with an awareness of the wider professional factors which are not always at the forefront of our minds.

Professional Regulation and Standards

The paramedic profession has been regulated since 2000; initially voluntarily, and originally with the Council for Professions Supplementary to Medicine (CPSM), becoming mandatory following the publication of the Health Professions Order (2001). In 2003, this Order was amended and gave rise to the formation of the Health Professions Council, which later became the Health and Care Professions Council (HCPC) we know today. The HCPC is responsible for the regulation of around 340,000 individual registrants across 16 professions, some of which are Allied Health Professions.

The following professions are regulated by the HCPC. Professions marked with an asterix are also recognised as Allied Health Professions (See Table 2.1 at the end of the chapter for more information about the HCPC professions):

1.   Arts therapists (includes dramatherapists and music therapists) *
2.   Biomedical scientists
3.   Chiropodists/podiatrists*
4.   Clinical scientists
5.   Dietitians*
6.   Hearing aid dispensers

7. Occupational therapists*

8. Operating department practitioners

9. Orthoptists*

10. Paramedics*

11. Physiotherapists*

12. Practitioner psychologists (e.g. clinical psychologists)

13. Prosthetists and orthotists*

14. Radiographers (therapeutic and diagnostic)*

15. Social workers in England

16. Speech and language therapists.*

The purpose of the HCPC, and in fact all nine healthcare regulators, such as the Nursing and Midwifery Council (NMC) and the General Medical Council (GMC), is to protect the public, not to serve its registrants. The HCPC along with the other eight regulators are overseen and scrutinised by the Professional Standards Authority, and all work to ensure that registrants uphold and follow the standards stated by each regulator.

All regulators publish their register. This allows members of the public to check if their healthcare professional is registered and/or subject to any conditions or sanctions. Importantly, employers can check whether their staff are registered, and work with regulators in cases involving their own staff members. Regulation should not be confused with membership of a professional body or a trades union, and the cost of registration is an essential aspect of professional practice.

The other key role of the professional regulator is to ensure that the protected titles associated with registered professions are not misused. This means that the regulator has the power to bring prosecutions against those who use protected titles without being registered. This is a very important aspect of registration and links closely to professional identity, which in turn provides further assurance to the public that the healthcare professionals providing their care are registered, authentic and practising to minimum standards.

The standards which are published by the HCPC should be read and understood by all registrants, as this gives vital information about the requirements of them as a healthcare professional. As well as published standards, the HCPC manage issues which arise involving registrants' fitness to practise, and will hear cases where standards have not been met, issuing sanctions where necessary.

Standards

The HCPC Standards include:

- Standards of proficiency for paramedics;

- Standards of conduct, performance and ethics;

- Standards for continuing professional development;

- Character;

- Health.

The full Standards are available to download from: www.hcpc-uk.org/
aboutregistration/standards

Fitness to Practise and Sanctions

Fitness to Practise (FTP) hearings are not intended to be punitive. In other words, the HCPC do not seek to apply a punishment considering acts or omissions, but where the issue is serious enough to warrant a punitive measure, suspension or striking from the register may be applied. The role of the FTP Panel is to judge whether the registrant is impaired, and therefore not fit to practise. The outcome of FTP hearings may conclude with no further action, but may lead to one of the following being applied:

- **Mediation**
  This is usually applied where the complainant's concerns are not fully resolved, but the hearing does not find against the registrant.

- **Caution**
  A caution may be applied to a registrant's record for between one and five years (three years being the most common), and recognises minor issues which have a very low risk of reoccurrence.

- **Conditions of practice**
  Conditions of practice may include a requirement to undertake further education and training to resolve the root cause of the issue, and is judged to have a low risk of reoccurrence. This may also include a restriction in practice, on its own, or in combination with a requirement to undertake further training.

- **Suspension**
  Suspension is for more serious concerns, but for which return to practice is appropriate after a period of time suspended. The period of suspension is a maximum of one year.

- **Striking off**
  The following is taken directly from the HCPC and highlights the nature of the consideration to striking a registrant from the register. These are less commonly related to clinical practice, and are associated with an incompatibility with professional practice.

  'Striking off is a sanction of last resort for serious, deliberate or reckless acts involving abuse of trust such as sexual abuse, dishonesty or persistent failure. Striking off should be used where there is no other way to protect the public,

for example, where there is a lack of insight, continuing problems or denial. An inability or unwillingness to resolve matters will suggest that a lower sanction may not be appropriate.'

(HCPC, 2015)

It is important to remember that the application of sanctions is primarily to ensure the public are assured that the professional is fit to practise, and also that the reputation of the profession is upheld.

Being Confident in Practice

In the context of decision making and being confident in practice, the statistics which relate to paramedic complaints and concerns made to the HCPC should be reflected upon as the reality of professional practice. Regulation means that you should not approach your professional role with fear of the regulator, instead the published standards should be used to guide you alongside your own values, morals and standards. We should remember that paramedics practise in extremely hostile environments, and therefore any lapses of judgement may be exacerbated by situational or other **human factors** (such as stress, fatigue or work intensity). Making sound decisions in all aspects of practice can provide the platform for defensible practice, and while paramedics are high in the league table of complaints to the regulator relative to the number of registrants, the profession features sixth in terms of concerns raised by the public. Self-referral at 31.7% is second only to social workers among HCPC registrants, and this may reflect the nature of some employee settings.

Professional Identity

Professional identity is defined by Ashforth, Harrison and Corley (2008) as the 'essential human desire to expand the self-concept to include connections with others and to feel a sense of belonging with a larger group'. This supports the definition by Ibarra (1999), which reflects on the 'relatively stable and enduring constellation of attributes, values, motives, and experiences in terms of which people define themselves in a professional role'. Your own perception of yourself as a paramedic is therefore very important. The way in which we demonstrate our collective values and behaviours is shaped by the standards published by our regulator, and is included in our curricula and practice guidance.

Professional identity can be drawn from a range of sources and cues, including shared values, common training, membership of a professional body, or even wearing a uniform. Identifying with your professional identity can create the same feelings of pride and community, similar to the way supporters of a football team behave, including how success and failure are managed collectively.

It concludes by saying that a strong professional identity can increase a professional's valuation of their role, which brings benefits, not only to the professional themselves but also to patients. How paramedics and other healthcare professionals view themselves is linked to behaviour in their practice settings, and how they work and communicate with colleagues. It is also important to reflect on how the image of paramedics as perceived by the public is perpetuated through professional practice, and challenged accordingly. Paramedics are not only working for ambulance services, and this is having an effect on professional identity and therefore there is a risk of some loss of identity where the green uniform isn't worn. This is a challenge for us as paramedics, but also a nice problem to have as paramedics are held in high regard by the public.

Biomedical Ethics

'Ethics is nothing else than reverence for life.'
(Albert Schweitzer, 1875–1965)

'A man without ethics is a wild beast loosed upon this world.'
(Albert Camus, 1913–1960)

Ethics in healthcare is a vast topic. It covers a wide range of areas and includes very complex models and concepts. It is led by academics from around the world, creating research and consensus that leads to better understanding of our human rights in all aspects of how we interact with the world around us. Ethics is simply the study and explanation of morality. It seeks to understand concepts such as the social consensus, examples of which include not stealing or murdering. Strong moral fibre is often assumed in healthcare professionals, and an understanding of key ethical principles can help them to understand and maintain their moral compass.

Putting the Patient First: Ethical Considerations in Practice

In healthcare, we are required through registration and regulation to practise ethically, and therefore this must become part of the decision-making process we use in our everyday practice when caring for patients. Considering how vast the subject is, it is important to develop a working understanding of the key concepts. The book *Principles of Biomedical Ethics* (Beauchamp and Childress, 2001) is arguably the most suitable place to begin understanding ethics for paramedics. There are four principles in the book, each of which can be explained and understood, and can be worked into our approach to patient encounters in order to promote the correct outcome. The discussion of each of the principles is intended to be at a high level and provide a broad-brush understanding linked to their application in practice.

Non-maleficence

Non-maleficence means *'first, do no harm.'*

It is accepted that some treatments have associated risks. Paramedics must ensure, therefore, that any treatments considered will provide greater benefit than risk to the patient, and are carried out without malice or other extrinsic reason. The benefits must outweigh the risks, and this is usually supported by clinical guidelines or other evidence-based drivers. Consideration must also be given to the risks of not withholding treatment, as the application of the treatment may also be harmful. For instance, where a patient has chosen not to be resuscitated due to the progression of their terminal illness, cardiopulmonary resuscitation (CPR) is most likely not to be successful. Any injuries (such as rib fractures) caused by CPR will be far more harmful and undignified in the context of trying to prevent the patient's inevitable demise.

Beneficence

A beneficent act is an act that is done for a patient's benefit. Beneficent acts may prevent harm or further harm, and/or can be used to improve the patient's situation.

For paramedics, undertaking resuscitation is the most obvious example of an act of **beneficence** as carrying out CPR may ultimately prevent death. Beneficence also includes more humanistic acts, such as preserving warmth and dignity, and helping reduce pain.

Beneficence is different from non-maleficence in that the act moves the patient away from harm and towards an improved situation. Think of it as the difference between pulling someone away from the edge of cliff, compared with pushing them off the cliff into a lake (if the latter was deemed to present less risk of overall harm, for example to escape a forest fire). In healthcare, encouraging patients to stop smoking or lose weight is a beneficent act as it is intended to prevent harm in the future.

Respect for Autonomy

Respecting autonomy means practising on the basis of the patient's wishes.

Autonomy, or **agency**, is the basic human right which protects the individual's right to self-determination, freedom, will etc. and in healthcare is the basis of patient-centred care. Many patients seen by paramedics have their autonomy suspended or diminished through injury or illness (i.e. head injury or dementia) and this makes decision making harder as, without prior knowledge of the patients' wishes, we may apply our own values and morals on the situation.

Justice

Justice is defined as the fair and equitable allocation of time and resources to promote the correct outcome for patients.

This concept is of particular interest and should be reflected on by paramedics on the basis that the traditional model of care often bookends patient contact ('one job at a time'). It could be argued that spending three hours with an older person who has fallen and is uninjured, but with whom the paramedic wishes to spend time, may be at the expense of someone with a life-threatening condition waiting longer for a response. The faller gets, in effect, 'too much' justice, and the patient waiting with the life-threatening condition gets less, or no justice. In the context of decision making, we should consider more carefully how we perceive ourselves as a resource, and how justly we self-allocate this to our patients.

In summary regarding ethics in practice, care is usually associated with a utilitarian ethical approach; the belief that doing the right thing increases overall 'good' consequences and is associated with the principle of beneficence (Beauchamp and Childress, 2001, p.166). Healthcare professionals are drawn naturally towards an intuitive approach to the essence of care. This translates well to the features of Kantian, **deontological ethics**, as the worth of the act is derived from evidence-based care protocols, but it has the potential to stifle ethical considerations when focusing on the patient as the end, rather than the means to an end. Jonathan Baron in his (2006) book *Against Bioethics* makes an interesting observation, which illustrates this point very effectively: '...*many moral intuitions are interesting psychological phenomena rather than windows into some sort of moral truth*'.

This section has barely scratched the surface of ethics, and is intended to cover some of the high-level concepts which can assist with decision making. There is a wealth of literature available, and the books and journal articles listed in the 'Ethics bibliography' at the end of this chapter should provide a useful start for further reading.

Patient-centred Care

In the modern NHS patients quite correctly have a voice, and this voice is aimed both at the shaping of services and at defining how healthcare encounters happen. In days gone by, healthcare was done *to* patients, rather than *with* them, and the enduring image of Jim Dale in *Carry on Doctor* forcibly having his underwear removed by Hattie Jacques typifies the importance of communication and consent. In biomedical ethics, the patient is paramount with Kantian, duty-based ethics stating that patients 'must always be the end in themselves and never a means to an end' (Kant, translated Bennett, 2008). In emergency care, and as paramedic practice has developed, the issue of consent has become ever more complex but increasingly better defined. The combination of an **action-biased** workforce and the notion of 'presumed consent' has led the need to move the patient to the centre, and ensure that they are fully informed of their care.

Patients are also extremely useful for decision makers, and quite apart from the ethical and value-based imperative, they often hold the key to their own illness or injury. History taking accounts for 90–95% of the diagnostic process, and while some warn of the 'bad historian', the clinician should apply competent processes which prevent the patient from failing to express their condition and impede a good diagnosis.

'Listen to your patient, he is telling you the diagnosis.'

(Sir William Osler, 1849–1919)

Consent is a vital aspect of promoting patient-centred care, and even more important in urgent, emergency and unscheduled care as the patient is more vulnerable and often less able to understand complex concepts due to pain or distress. The effective decision maker must of course be decisive and present a confident front in order for the patient to be reassured as much as possible. But the balance must be struck between rote, paternalistic care delivery and care which is delivered in partnership with the patient, and wherever possible that care is delivered with the full informed consent, or at least assent, of the patient.

Patient-centred care is much more than a modern buzzword in healthcare, and can be considered in the following analogy.

A woman takes her car to the local garage complaining that the car is making a funny noise. She says she thinks the exhaust has a hole in it. 'Of course it's got a hole in it, that's where the fumes come out, love!' the mechanic says. 'No, a new hole. It's making a rasping noise, and I need some advice'. The mechanic explains that he can change the exhaust if she would like. The woman isn't a mechanic and does not have the expertise to know whether the exhaust can be repaired. She is worried that this might be an unnecessary expense, and the experience is making her anxious and upset.

Imagine if that was in a healthcare encounter. The woman knows that something is wrong and it might be simple and easy to treat. In the case above, had the mechanic used the equivalent of patient-centred care, the scenario would have been very different. How many times have you seen a patient's needs dismissed because the patient wasn't put first, perhaps because they couldn't express their concerns? Remember, the patient must only ever be the end, and never a means to an end.

Another example, seen in Chapter 1, was that of the paramedics who took a patient to hospital, despite the fact that the patient clearly could have been cared for in the community, because they knew they could get themselves a cup of tea at the hospital. The patient is paramount. The patient's experience of care often affects their outcome and recovery. Always base your decision making about the patient on what is best for them.

Confidentiality

One of the fundamental aspects of the relationship between clinician and patient is the bond of confidentiality. Patients' personal information must be protected. There are very limited circumstances where not respecting a patient's confidentiality can be considered, such as where a crime has been committed.

NHS England has published a confidentiality policy which includes the following statement:

> 'All employees working in the NHS are bound by a legal duty of confidence to protect personal information they may come into contact with during the course of their work. This is not just a requirement of their contractual responsibilities but also a requirement within the common law duty of confidence and the Data Protection Act (1998). It is also a requirement within the NHS Care Record Guarantee, produced to assure patients regarding the use of their information.'
>
> (NHS England, 2016)

This passage highlights the importance of confidentiality, both in terms of protecting patients and the public, but also in relation to the legislative requirements of upholding the security of personal data detailed in the Data Protection Act. Maintaining confidentiality is an active process. Clinicians should include, within their decision-making process, the steps they will consider to protect patients' data.

The HCPC publishes guidance for registrants, which includes the following principles:

- *Take all reasonable steps to keep information about service users safe.*
- *Get the service user's informed consent if you are passing on their information, and get express consent, in writing, if you are using the information for reasons which are not related to providing care or services for the service user.*
- *Disclose identifiable information only if it is absolutely necessary. When it is necessary, only disclose the minimum amount necessary.*
- *Tell service users when you have disclosed their information (if this is practical and possible).*
- *Keep appropriate records of disclosure.*
- *Keep up to date with relevant law and good practice.*
- *If appropriate, ask for advice from colleagues, professional bodies, unions, legal professionals or us.*
- *Make your own informed decisions about disclosure and be able to justify them.*

(HCPC, 2012)

This guidance from the HCPC must be read and understood in order to achieve a minimum standard in applying confidentiality to clinical practice. There are still many pitfalls which may not be considered directly by paramedics in practice, the most common one being the use of social media.

The use of social media by healthcare professionals to support CPD and inter-collegiate communication is growing and this can be very positive. However, there is also a rise in the practice of recording and sharing experiences through these platforms as an extension of healthcare professionals' private lives. The decision-making processes used in diagnosis and patient management can be applied to choices regarding social media. For example, the decision to photograph the scene of a road accident and post to social media may provide a point of interest for friends and family. But if a patient is identified as a result of this, or information is deemed to have been shared inappropriately or otherwise in line with the responsibilities of the registrant, the consequences may be significant. Sanctions have been applied in several cases in recent years.

Competence and Confidence in Practice

The theme, which appears throughout this book, is the link between competency and confidence in practice, linked to the need to practise defensibly, rather than defensively. Reflecting on how good decision making can increase the confidence in the decisions being made, and the processes described as a suggested way of improving how decisions are made, which itself becomes a competency, just leaves confidence as a concept without a clear definition.

Competency: '*an important skill that is needed to do a job.*'

Confidence: '*the quality of being certain of your abilities or of having trust in people, plans, or the future.*'

(Cambridge Dictionary, 2017)

Unlike confidence, competency can be viewed as qualitative as well as quantitative. The acquisition of skills may be binary (able or unable to) and can be assessed accordingly as evidence of ability. Alternatively, it may emerge over a period of time along a 'novice to expert' path. Can we assess confidence in the same way? How can we remind ourselves that we either are confident, or should be confident?

Confidence is a lived experience, and is a psychological condition, which is hard to assess compared to psychomotor skills (**suturing**, for instance). It may be felt by the individual and/or observed by others.

- *After that last resus, she has really lost her confidence.*
- *I have never been confident when dealing with children.*
- *Passing the exam really improved my confidence.*

Being confident has a positive impact on patients, and no patient wants to be cared for by a healthcare professional who lacks confidence and displays this outwardly. Confidence in practice may be linked to culture, local policy, management style, or a host of other issues, which may be directly or indirectly linked to clinical practice. Approaching problems with confidence is important, and learning what you can be confident about is a way of overcoming the anxieties which can impact negatively on your time in the workplace. The notion of **epistemological** self-confidence – a belief in what you know and what you do – is certainly something to aim for if you are starting from a position of weak confidence. It is certainly preferable to over-confidence or complacency.

Confidence in practice grows over time, but can also diminish following events and the risk of a poor outcome. Confidence can be optimised through reflection, self-awareness, consolidated experience, and willingness to learn from error. Healthcare is developing a more just culture in which learning can drive continuous improvements in care. Building and maintaining confidence is on a gradient, which may differ depending on the type of patient you are seeing (trauma vs medical for example). Ultimately, though, confidence colours your experience in practice, and so should be seen as something to work on and develop in the same way you develop your other skills.

Professional Insight

In Chapter 4, we will discuss some of the biases and fallacies that beset the human condition – such as the issue of unconscious incompetence (I don't know what I don't know). This in turn links closely to professional insight; knowing what you know about yourself and how this may affect the care you give. It is subtly different from technical competence and is associated with more complex considerations, including the ego, which impacts on how you feel and function. Conditioning yourself to have a healthy scepticism of your own ability is vitally important (see 'The Summit of Mount Stupid' in Chapter 3) and will work to support your practice and protect your patient.

Insight is defined as awareness and perception; understanding and comprehension, and perspicacity, and infers a deep cognitive view on how things really are. An astute self-assessment of how well you perform can lead to far better decisions, and should be seen in a very positive (rather than a defeatist) way. This can inform how delegation takes place at the patient's side – you may assess your own ability to achieve difficult IV access in comparison to a colleague who has previously demonstrated to you that they are more proficient, and therefore more likely to succeed. Parking your own ego and focusing on the logical argument can provide a greater sense of achievement in how care is ultimately delivered. This requires professional insight and, to some degree, personal sacrifice.

Professional insight has a very real utility in the presence of error and harm, and how you behave and respond to situations that have a poor outcome. Those with strong professional insight are the first to raise their hand where things go wrong and are less likely to cover up their mistakes, choosing instead to learn from them. Where professional insight is strongest, the decision to share the event with colleagues in an action learning group or peer review may happen.

Summary

Professional practice extends beyond the confines of the patient/clinician interface, and the acts, omissions, judgements and behaviours of all healthcare professionals must be considered in the context of your professional identity and standards. Registered healthcare practice also extends beyond periods of time at work, and while this may appear overbearing, it is a reflection of the trust and faith society has on those with the skills and aptitude to provide care for patients. For paramedics, that care is often provided at a time for the patient when their needs are at the most acute, and where the environment is most hostile – usually figuratively speaking, but often also practically speaking.

Professional considerations are unlikely to be explicitly included in guidelines and protocols, and can exist in the murky areas between best practice, legislation, humanity, and morality. Navigating professional issues can be made clearer through the decision you make if you take a moment to consider these in the context of the practice dilemma being managed. Your developing decision-making skills will help you maintain patient safety, and will prompt you to think critically rather than accept what you may have unknowingly processed in the past.

Conclusion

The end of this chapter concludes the concepts and principles which together can form a model for you to use and develop in practice in order to make safe and defensible decisions for your clinical encounters with your patients. As with many things in life, the processes described are not the only way to achieve the goal of becoming a safe decision maker, and you may want to keep reading perhaps more deeply into the field of behaviour and psychology, or look more broadly at other decision-making models which are most compatible with your particular approach.

The purpose of this whole book is to open up lines of enquiry within oneself in order to face the main issue, which befalls human beings who are asked to do complex tasks: we weren't designed to do any of this! The conflict between the old part of the human brain (which is impulsive and rash and has the loudest voice), and the new part (which is slow and deliberate) is what causes bad decisions and bad outcomes. It can be tamed and managed, and you can improve the responsiveness of your new brain by using techniques which encourage you to challenge what you think you have heard or seen.

The days of using only experience and intuition, with the safety net of being able to move patients to another professional or care setting every time, are over. Many patients have manageable presentations in the community, and the way decisions are made needs to be done with a wider range of cues and considerations. These considerations must be analysed critically – sometimes using scepticism and cynicism – but always focused on doing the right thing. The next chapter will look in more detail at critical thinking as a foundation for approaching the management of challenges in practice.

Reflective Exercises

- Ethical considerations are extremely important for patients in clinical practice. Pick one of the principles of biomedical ethics and reflect on a case you have dealt with, applying the key considerations for that principle. Test the impact on your decision making.

- Consider the importance of professional insight in your own practice. Test your own levels of humility and ego, reflecting on errors you have made in the past. How can your insight drive improvements to your knowledge and skill without diminishing your confidence?

- Select one of the published regulatory standards documents from the HCPC website. Reflect on the importance of it in relation to the function of the regulator. Why is this important, and what do paramedics need to understand as an intrinsic aspect of their practice?

Ethics Bibliography

- Beauchamp, T.L. and Childress, J.F. (2001) *Principles of Biomedical Ethics*. 5th ed. Oxford: Oxford University Press.

- Hope, T. (2004) *Medical Ethics: A Very Short Introduction*. Oxford: Oxford University Press.

- Murdoch, I. (1971). *The Sovereignty of Good*. London: Routledge.

- Runzheimer, J. and Johnson Larsen, L. (2011) *Medical Ethics for Dummies*. Hoboken, USA: Wiley.

Health Profession	Protected Titles	Approximate Number of Registrants (2016)
Arts therapists	Art psychotherapist Art therapist Dramatherapist Music therapist	3,741
Biomedical scientists	Biomedical scientist	22,386
Chiropodists/podiatrists	Chiropodist Podiatrist	13,111
Clinical scientists	Clinical scientist	5,442
Dietitians	Dietitian	8,828

Health Profession	Protected Titles	Approximate Number of Registrants (2016)
Hearing aid dispensers	Hearing aid dispenser	2,451
Occupational therapists	Occupational therapist	36,844
Operating department practitioners	Operating department practitioner	12,856
Orthoptists	Orthoptist	1,406
Paramedics	Paramedic	22,778
Physiotherapists	Physical therapist Physiotherapist	51,199
Practitioner psychologists (e.g. Clinical psychologists)	Clinical psychologist Counselling psychologist Educational psychologist Forensic psychologist Health psychologist Occupational psychologist Practitioner psychologist Registered psychologist Sport and exercise psychologist	21,670
Prosthetists and orthotists	Orthotist Prosthetist	1,037
Radiographers	Diagnostic radiographer Radiographer Therapeutic radiographer	31,292
Social workers in England	Social worker	93,962
Speech and language therapists	Speech and language therapist Speech therapist	15,424

Table 2.1: *List of professions regulated by the Health and Care Professions Council*

3 The Evolution of the Paramedic as a Critical Thinker

Chapter Objectives

This chapter will cover:

- Critical thinking in everyday life;
- Approach to critical thinking in paramedic practice;
- Decision making, values and healthcare practice;
- Barriers to critical thinking;
- Intuition and experience in critical thinking;
- Decision Point Management: a critical thinking tool;
- Summing up: moving from 'what' to 'why'.

Caution!

This chapter will introduce the process of challenging yourself in terms of what you believe when making decisions, and how this process needs time and deliberation (**System 2 thinking**) (Kahneman, 2011). In paramedic practice, there are often situations where immediate action is required. It is this ability – among the wider skill set of paramedics – which helps define what paramedics do for patients in high pressure situations.

The intention of this chapter and the following chapters is to allow a decision-making acumen to develop which promotes better outcomes, but care must be taken to avoid delaying treatment when there is not the time to deliberate (**System 1 thinking**) (Kahneman, 2011). Do not let these new concepts prevent you from acting decisively in an emergency.

Approach to Critical Thinking in Everyday Life and Paramedic Practice

As we human beings go through life, we may impose on ourselves (or accept) concepts which we believe to be true, accurate and correct. Whether this is a subjective opinion on what colours we consider to be appealing, or objective views which may or may not be factually correct, we tend to favour one thing over another for a variety of reasons. This is part of having a human personality. Sharing views and opinions helps us form and maintain relationships. For example, supporting a particular football team (regardless of how often they lose) enables us to feel part of a group. The wide variety of factors which joins tribes together also has the power to divide, as our preferences in areas such as values, morals, ethics and tolerance are often highly subjective. Where decisions are left unchallenged, and never subject to reflection, they can become entirely intuitive. Or they can be based on cultural beliefs or tribal behaviours, and the level of influence or bias entirely missed. Some subjective tribal beliefs are harmless, but others lead to decisions being made which may be highly unethical. Biomedical ethics is discussed in more detail in Chapter 2, but the following example highlights an extreme instance of human vulnerabilities in thought and decision making where **group-think** and influence is strong.

Example: The KKK

The Ku Klux Klan (KKK) is an organisation whose stock-in-trade is exclusion by dint of race. It is arguably one of the most evil organisations on the planet (accepting that competition in this area is sadly demonstrably and historically fierce). To those who subscribe to the KKK way of thinking, the cruelty demonstrated in the 1950s and 60s by Klansmen is not seen as a bleak period of their history. Rather, it is their halcyon era where their beliefs resonated with far more people than they do now. Importantly, and considering how we are influenced or even coerced, those born into a KKK community, and who have no moral frame of reference allowing the formation of a reasonable balanced alternative view, may never rationalise (or even consider) the intent to divide and discriminate against others outside of their community or racial group. While this is in no way justification, and certainly does not condone, for them it probably seems normal and natural to think and behave the way they do. Similarly, they may find the more common, and socially acceptable, counterpoise irrational.

Clearly this is an extreme example, but this kind of intractable viewpoint is by no means unique in human history. It demonstrates that human beings are capable of becoming blinkered to the wider ranges of choice and judgement, and some are prone to being influenced and misled into adopting narrow and flawed beliefs which are wildly at odds with the majority of reasonable members of society. Consider the Stanford University Experiment undertaken in 1971, where students adopted randomly assigned roles as either prisoners or guards. Within six days, the experiment was abandoned due to the behaviours of the 'guards' – students – who only a few days previously were mild-mannered young undergraduates. The prevailing culture provided a snapshot of how humans can react if the social norms are interrupted and group-think becomes established. These were intelligent people, and it is fascinating to reflect on how quickly the landscape changed and how reasonable decisions stopped being made. How can the culture in healthcare settings affect how we make decisions? Do we have 'bad apples' or 'bad barrels'?

> *How we went about testing these questions and what we found may astound you. Our planned two-week investigation into the psychology of prison life had to be ended after only six days because of what the situation was doing to the college students who participated. In only a few days, our guards became sadistic and our prisoners became depressed and showed signs of extreme stress.*
>
> (Professor Philip G. Zimbardo in Haney et al., 1973)

The links between these examples and patient care and clinical practice may seem distant, but there may be some aspects to your practice that you consider normal and mundane, and for which you have never been challenged. These may be actually quite outdated, outmoded or dangerous, and may have arisen through subliminal learning or within a small social group, manifested as 'group-think' or tribal behaviour. The examples given serve to illustrate that deeply rooted beliefs about what is correct or accurate may have been imparted in such a way that they may never be challenged. This is part of the human condition, so we do need to broaden our horizons in order to learn and make decisions. In the healthcare setting this takes on even greater level of importance as the ever-evolving and developing evidence base means that challenging preconceptions is vital in preventing harm to patients.

The fact is that we are all capable of being influenced into unreasonable, irrational thoughts, acts and beliefs. Most are not harmful, but are equally irrational – such as buying lottery tickets, fear of flying regardless of the prevailing statistics, or listening to Coldplay (sorry, but I did say we are prone to subjectivity). The important principle of challenging preconceptions may, in the healthcare setting, alter some outcomes for the better for patients. Looking at the way humanity can be so easily influenced is important to highlight that we can all make poor decisions where we fail to critically appraise information and instead allow ourselves to 'go with the flow'. We will now try to understand why this happens, in the hope of ensuring it doesn't happen to us.

Decision Making, Values and Healthcare Practice

As previously discussed, we are not inherently driven to constantly question ourselves. This means that we can easily become entrenched in our ways and views. Regardless of this, these factors combine to form us as a person – for better or worse. The beliefs and experiences we accumulate, along with knowledge and learned behaviours, coalesce to become our personality. This works very nicely for the most part. Friendships are made on the basis of commonality of thought and purpose, values are defined and reinforced, and ultimately what we believe is true becomes as everyday as the impulse to reach for the light switch when you walk into a darkened room. Critical thinking is a process for challenging, where appropriate and/or necessary, these entrenched truths – the **heuristically** implanted notions which are stored as fact but which can betray you – leading to a place where subjectivity can be replaced with objectivity where necessary. Clearly, this works best where something is equivocal rather than an opinion that has limited impact on others. For example, some people are moved by certain pieces of modern art and sculpture, while others think they are just piles of bricks or unmade beds. The point is that it doesn't really matter in that case as the subjectivity requires no establishment of fact and the beauty is, of course, in the eye of the beholder. When this is transferred to a health encounter, any subjectivity which isn't robustly tested may be actively harmful, and this is in essence the cornerstone of evidence-based medicine (NICE, 2016). As paramedics we are bound, through regulatory standards, to practise according to the best evidence (HCPC, 2016). Imagine, for example, if you decided to assume that all children's rashes were caused by a simple viral infection, rather than a bacterial illness, and refused to examine any evidence that might contradict this. If your diagnostic preference went unchallenged, it would ultimately lead to poor outcomes for some patients. The basis of what we observe or test for as clinicians should be treated with suspicion and doubt until it can be reduced down to fact (or as near to fact as possible). We will now look at the process of turning 'what' to 'why' and how following this mantra can provide a really simple method for ensuring that each encounter you have with patients is approached in such a way as to ensure you can test your skills and knowledge and come up with the best answer for the presentation you are facing.

Exercise: Turning WHAT into WHY

Please look at the image below:

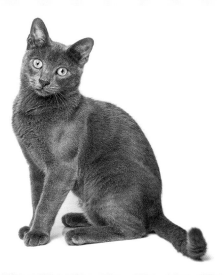

Figure 3.1: Object identification

Can you identify the subject of the picture? Of course, you can, but all you have done is say 'what' it is. Now look again and ask 'why' it is what you think it is. Challenge yourself to find features that are unequivocally associated with a cat to the point where you may only be happy to say it's a cat because it has sufficient individual factors which satisfies you that the picture has the 'essence of cat'. This activity is a simplified test of turning 'what' into 'why' and is not as easy as you first think. Critically analysing each factor and finding out that most of the identifiable features could actually make this a dog or a goat should make you think more about other things you think are true!

This will be useful later in the chapter, I promise!

The rest of this chapter will focus on raising the profile of critical thinking, and analytical processes as an intrinsic part of your decision-making acumen and which can greatly assist your practice. By understanding the basic concepts of critical thinking you will be able to think with more clarity, be more observant and learn to exploit more information. You will become sufficiently skilled to be able to build arguments which will form your dynamic responses to challenges, or to form hypotheses in more complex situations. Building an argument with yourself to prove what you think you are seeing or experiencing is key to moving towards a more robust processing model, along with other stratagems such as **shared decision making**. Later chapters look at **hypothetico-deduction** as an appropriate model in paramedic practice, as the development of the **hypothesis** requires a process too. This is where critical thinking has a strong place in your arsenal. Many situations are linked with apparently unequivocal answers – self-evident circumstances, situations or pathologies (equivalent to identifying a cat) – and it's these situations where dynamic analysis can be rapidly used to ensure a healthy level of distrust and scepticism in a positive way to ensure what you are seeing, hearing or experiencing is true. For example, think of times when you have to cross a road which is usually busy, but now it has no traffic flowing because of an incident. The presence of an empty road suggests it's safe to cross. All you have done is identify the 'what'; *the empty road* with no apparent dangers. By *not* trusting your instinct, you quickly ask *why* is it safe and consider that the expected norms have been altered, such as the risk/potential for other emergency vehicles travelling on the wrong side of the road to access the scene. This is not a deductive process, rather it's a dynamic process which requires critical thinking to ensure that the reasons to act are quickly assessed rather than viewed as the truth – 'before I act, can I trust my instinct?' Many texts include decision making as merely an aspect of critical thinking, and this is true, but only in the dynamic sense. Arguably, in clinical practice, critical thinking cross-cuts decision making and has a utility in many stages of information processing, categorisation and diagnosis. Put simply, critically appraise what you see balanced with the other pieces of information you have; act upon it quickly when you need to, and use it to shape hypothesis when more consideration is needed.

The intention to think critically is easy to do but making it part of your everyday processes needs attention and purposeful practice otherwise you may let your guard down, and this will affect your decision making.

Barriers to Critical Thinking

Critical thinking is about considering how you think. It must be practised, like any task which becomes a skill. Critical thinking is learned ability; few people have these skills innately suggesting that practice will improve your access to this ability and increase its usefulness. In this way, the initial clumsiness you may experience will diminish with time. All new skills feel alien and difficult, but that shouldn't stop you from persevering. In *Bounce*, the author Matthew Syed (2011) discusses being able to become an expert following 10,000 hours of 'purposeful practice'. If you are learning to play table tennis or the guitar, you may be fortunate to find a few hours each week to practise, but decades of dedication will be necessary if you are to achieve expertise. Critical thinking, however, can be practised in virtually every waking moment, and certainly during the working week. Someone practising table tennis for 37.5 hours each week would take just over five years to achieve 10,000 hours of practice to become an expert table tennis player, but in critical thinking if you apply your craft to every waking hour you would achieve this in less than two years.

Clearly, the idea of highlighting periods of defined, purposeful practice is an exaggeration, and in reality once you have moved on from the initial clumsy period associated with any new skill you will not consciously switch the process on and off. In due course, you may not be aware to the level where you could retrospectively identify each time you thought critically. It is, however, important that you are always aware you are *able* to think critically so you can be aware where you may not be thinking critically. As this awareness diminishes you will need to retain an awareness of where you may be prone to not thinking critically, and there are plenty of barriers to practising and using critical thinking. It is important therefore to identify these threats so you can recognise when these extrinsic factors are interfering with your practice. Before reading on, let's do a quick exercise.

Critical Thinking Exercise: Making Links and Association Bias

Read the following nursery rhyme:

Humpty Dumpty

Humpty Dumpty sat on a wall,
Humpty Dumpty had a great fall.
All the King's horses and all the King's men
Couldn't put Humpty together again.

And the following recipe:

The Ultimate Meringue

4 large organic egg whites, at room temperature
115g caster sugar
115g icing sugar

What immediately springs to mind as connecting these two quite disparate things – a nursery rhyme and a recipe?

The obvious answer is of course *eggs*, and why wouldn't you make that link – unless of course you were thinking critically. Perhaps go back and read the two passages again and look more carefully at what you are reading, and challenge your instinctive, intuitive response. Park your preconceptions and answer the questions '*what is the link?*' and '*is there a link, and if so why?*' The answer is that there is no actual evidential link whatsoever. There is nothing to state that Humpty Dumpty was an egg, and the origin of the nursery rhyme suggests no clear intent for the subject to be thought of as an egg. We are all aware of the nursery rhyme, and the image of Humpty Dumpty as an egg has been etched into our consciousness to a point where the absence of the word 'egg' has become entirely detached from our belief that Humpty Dumpty was in fact an egg. Moreover, it's hard to imagine anything other than an egg when you hear the words Humpty Dumpty. We must always assume there is a link until we can prove there isn't, and in clinical care we must look for the red flags or other critical factors until we can prove there aren't any.

In yet another (albeit ground-based) aviation analogy, airport security staff looking at bags passing through the x-ray scanner do not glance at each image and assume there is nothing sinister, they ask the vital question every time a bag passes – and it's the same question you must ask yourself '*where is the bomb*' (Rosenorn-Lanng, 2014, p.1).

It is also worth noting for completeness that there is a vegan recipe for meringue which uses chickpea brine – aquafaba – instead of egg whites. Where more information is available, linking Humpty Dumpty and meringue may elicit no evidence of eggs at all!

Now we have worked through a very specific exercise where we may have been betrayed by a longstanding childhood belief, let's look at some other barriers to critical thinking. The contents in the following table are arguably the cornerstones of the barriers to critical thinking, and were developed by Dr Richard Paul and Dr Linda Elder (The Foundation for Critical Thinking, 2001). These five headings resonate with healthcare practice and support the argument that we as humans are flawed thinkers due to competing personality traits, influences, biases, and fallacies.

Remember, if you cannot think critically you cannot develop hypotheses which are essential to the more complex decision-making processes covered later in the book.

Table 3.1 is taken from *The Miniature Guide to Critical Thinking: Concepts and Tools* by Paul and Elder (2001).

'It's true because I believe it.'	**Innate egocentrism**
	I assume that what I believe is true even though I have never questioned the basis for many of my beliefs.
	Example: *'You can never give a patient too much oxygen.'*
'It's true because we believe it.'	**Innate sociocentrism**
	I assume that the dominant beliefs of the groups to which I belong are true even though I have never questioned the basis for those beliefs.
	Example: *'We have always done it this way at my ambulance station.' (Tribal behaviour)*
'It's true because I want to believe it.'	**Innate wish fulfilment**
	I believe what 'feels good', what does not require me to change my thinking in any significant way, what does not require me to admit I have been wrong.
	Example: *'It's fine to stay with every patient as long as I like. I don't believe it affects other patients or my colleagues.'*
'It's true because I have always believed it.'	**Innate self-validation**
	I have a strong desire to maintain beliefs I have long held, even though I have not seriously considered the extent to which those beliefs are justified by the evidence.
	Example: *'I was shown this method on my Technician course 20 years ago – why should I do it differently now?'*
'It's true because it is in my selfish interest to believe it.'	**Innate selfishness**
	I believe whatever justifies my getting more power, or personal advantage even though those beliefs are not grounded in sound reasoning or evidence.
	Example: *'I don't believe that any patient wouldn't want to be resuscitated, so I carry out advanced life support on every patient regardless. It's my professional registration at stake after all!'*

Table 3.1: *Breaking down critical thinking*

Egotism vs Humility

We all like to believe that we are competent, and that our knowledge and skills are of a high standard. It is important – perhaps even vital – to park any preconceptions you may have (or may develop) about a situation due to your position within the care team, such as rank or seniority. There are many examples of where ego and a lack of insight leads to poor interpersonal relationships and which cause harm. While more and more clinical encounters managed by paramedics happen outside of the traditional ambulance crew configuration, critical thinking can and should occur within any relationship during an encounter (Professional/Carer, Professional/Family, Professional/Professional etc.), and perhaps the most important relationship to work on is between you and your ego. Building an argument with yourself is a crucial skill, and much harder than being challenged by a colleague.

Much of the work to improve safety in aviation has its origins in managing human error and human flaws (such as ego and hierarchy) and these traits are key aspects of what are known as **human factors** (see Chapter 4) – the aspects of human nature which can influence decisions and outcomes (Rosenorn-Lanng, 2014). The Tenerife air disaster, which occurred on 27 March 1977, typifies a situation where a lack of insight (and ego) displayed by the pilot of the KLM Boeing 747, and the fear shown by the first officer who chose not to challenge his decision, led to the death of over 500 people on the runway that day. The following passage is taken from the Spanish Authority's investigation report:

> **5.2. Authority in the Cockpit.** *Although nothing abnormal can be deduced from the CVR (Cockpit Voice Recorder), the fact exists that a co-pilot not very experienced with [Boeing] 747s was flying with one of the pilots of greatest prestige in the company who was, moreover, KLM's chief flying instructor and who had certified him fit to be a crew member for this type of aeroplane. In case of doubt, these circumstances could have induced the co-pilot not to ask any questions and to assume that this captain was always right.*
>
> (Air Line Pilots' Association, 1977)

Today, any member of flight crew can challenge the captain, and this approach has, with varying success, transferred to healthcare. In the operating theatre setting, for example, any clinician – doctor, nurse, operating department practitioner – is encouraged to speak out where they perceive a problem. This has led to the avoidance of serious errors such as the removal of incorrect limbs or organs.

The journey to becoming a good decision maker and critical thinker does involve understanding our own frailties in terms of how we perceive ourselves, and this requires the emergence of humility over ego, and an assessment of our own true belief in our own abilities. We tend to overstate our abilities (see Chapter 5 – the Dunning-Kruger Effect – Dunning & Kruger, 1999). This can lead to our ego or **sociocentricity** (group-think) to diminish our objectivity. You can link concepts such as the Dreyfus Model (1980) used by Benner (1984) in *From Novice to Expert* to assist with your own introspection and build on the balance between ego and humility. In simple terms, the more of a novice you are, the more humility you should display (see Figure 3.2). It is fine to know that you don't know something rather than to guess and cause your patient harm.

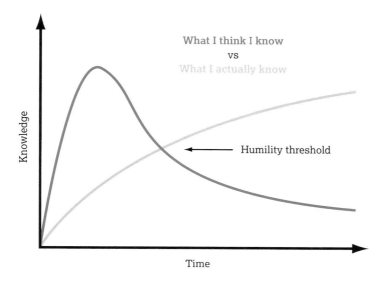

Figure 3.2: *Mount Stupid – Knowledge vs Experience. Graphic by Joseph F. Paris Jr. https://josephparis.me/my-articles/lessons-from-mt-stupid/ Used with Permission.*

Selfishness: Emotional Influence and Personal Values

Clinicians must make decisions with patients and respect their views, beliefs and wishes. It is not uncommon to come across a patient who has full **mental capacity** but makes an apparently bad decision about their own care. Thinking back to the beliefs we hold, and how we develop these beliefs, you may find it distressing for someone to decide that they do not wish for their treatable condition to be cured because you may have been brought up in a particular way, or have developed strong views throughout life – perhaps in response to a similar life event.

Emotional drivers and values are personal to the individual, and we cannot make good decisions which are contrary to the patient's wishes, however unreasonable these may be. You may find yourself concerned that if you leave the patient at home to die, their relatives will complain, and this will lead to disciplinary action. The experience of feeling these fears and other emotions is very real and can cloud one's judgement. Therefore, it is important to learn to understand how to suspend your own beliefs in order to uphold the patient's wishes, and how this can lead to the decision made being correct rather than imposed based on your values, and therefore wrong.

Other Important Barriers to Critical Thinking

If you search the internet or academic sources using the term *'Barriers to Critical Thinking'* you will be able to find almost every aspect of human consciousness and personality trait that can get in the way of critiquing what you see. There are many academic texts which focus on specific areas such as building arguments, challenging experts, and negotiating, but in the context of healthcare decision making, focus should be on those factors which actively or passively promote doing the best for the patient, rather than perhaps the more esoteric concepts.

Table 3.2 below can be used to explore the more specific barriers to critical thinking and are drawn from the list taken from Denis Korn (2016).

When you review these terms, you may recognise some of the traits in yourself and others, and this can be alarming. Healthcare professionals may view themselves as entirely rational and intelligent beings. The thought that superstition or wishful thinking could enter a health encounter is somewhat alien, but these two examples are seen often in hospitals. Many nurses will open the window in a room where a patient has died – a superstition. Our innate desire to hope our patients have a good outcome is often wishful thinking, but we do it anyway. These are fairly harmless barriers to critical thinking, but where concepts like pride, denial, and infallibility are introduced, these present very real threats to patients and must be better understood.

Barrier	Example
Absolutism	This barrier assumes that there are no exceptions, and that rules or tenets are absolute. Some ethical considerations are absolutist, and may link to concepts such as human rights. Where appropriate, this is a positive concept, but in healthcare it may be too constrained and lead to poor decisions being made – particularly where based on an incorrect belief (e.g. taking every patient to hospital to avoid ever getting a complaint).
An over-reliance on feelings	Intuition is an example of over-reliance on feelings, and is often considered as 'gut feelings', or actions resulting from emotional influence rather than scientific or deductive enquiry.
Cognitive dissonance	Conflict or inconsistency in thoughts and beliefs. In healthcare, this may be manifested as variations in practice – perhaps where provision of care is different for some patients due to factors such as confidence, competence or ignorance.

Barrier	Example
Conformism	This is mostly commonly a manifestation displayed where guidelines are applied in a rote way, and used as rules which are applied to the letter and to the exclusion of other considerations.
Debilitating fear and uncertainty	In the paramedic practice setting, this barrier is associated with fear of being disciplined at work or being struck off by the regulator. Conversely, this fear may create worse decisions and provide inferior care for the patient; similar to the absolutist approach, taking every patient to hospital in order to avoid criticism, thus failing to make proper decisions.
Denial	This may be one of the more troubling barriers to critical thinking, and in our practice settings may be experienced in situations where a procedure has been carried out to a poor standard, but the clinician convinces him or herself that it is fine – perhaps a cannula which won't flush which should be removed and another attempt made.
Disturbing one's comfort	Allowing ourselves to operate in the 'comfort zone' may lead to a lack of challenge, reflection and insight. Our comfort should be disturbed in order to think critically and avoid a stagnated approach.
Fear of being wrong or face-saving	Who wants to be wrong? One of the main demonstrable traits of an active learner and critical thinker is the lack of fear of being wrong and working collaboratively to ensure the correct outcome. Some people will not try in order to avoid failing (for instance, never taking a driving test in case you fail).
Fear of change or an unwillingness to change	We have discussed several times throughout this book the changing face of healthcare and the constantly changing patient profiles and behaviours.
Lack of discernment	Discernment is at the heart of critical thinking – considering and deciding on the quality or veracity of evidence or arguments. If you avoid discernment, you are not a critical thinker.
Lack of humility	Linked very closely to egocentrism, a lack of humility (often manifested as arrogance or overplaying experience) leads to poorly structured decision making and intuitive judgements. Humility is a trait associated with confident people with smaller egos who reflect on their practice.

Barrier	Example
Narrow-mindedness or closed-mindedness	How often have we heard a colleague say they don't believe in something? In healthcare, the evidence base changes often and we must keep pace. Fixing on concepts which become outmoded is an example of where narrow-mindedness can impede critical thinking.
Peer pressure	If you subscribe to the notion that there are no bad apples – only bad barrels – the influence of peer pressure could exist in a positive or negative way. Peer pressure implies conformity to an established norm or a culture which prevents challenge. Remember that history tells us following orders is no defence. Neither is citing peer-pressure.
Pride	A dent in your pride is rarely fatal, so don't approach practice with the intention of preserving it at all costs. Being wrong is important and allows reflection and learning. It's better to experience a loss of pride than have to explain to a coroner why you acted as you did.
Sociocentrism or **ethnocentrism**	In the same way we associate peer-pressure as a barrier to critical thinking, group-think and cultural beliefs to which you subscribe to (or to which you are expected to subscribe) also diminishes effective reasoning.
Stereotyping	This is much rarer now due to the work undertaken across health and social care to recognise diversity and vulnerabilities. On occasion though, some patients are unfairly grouped and stereotyped based on factors which are not directly relevant. For instance, frequent callers/attenders may be dismissed as a nuisance, leading to their issues not being resolved. Critically appraising why patients return time and again will promote the correct decision for their onward care.
Wishful thinking	'I am sure this will be fine'. You aren't sure, and this is not a good basis for resolving an episode of patient care. Remember that most errors and poor judgements don't cause harm and go undetected. One of the core tenets of this book is to remove doubt, and avoid wishful thinking.

Table 3.2: Barriers to critical thinking

Intuition and Experience in Critical Thinking

There is a theme throughout this book which suggests that intuition is a bad thing if not closely monitored and sparingly used, and that experience is only as good as the time spent reflecting and consolidating it after the event. What this does *not* mean is that the acquisition of experiences should not lead to faster access to problem solving in parallel with progressing towards expertise. Intuition should always be critically appraised where time permits whenever a similar situation occurs (such as the approach to the patient in cardiac arrest, where protocol determines action and action is informed by situational awareness). Where you clearly know what to do in a situation, that shouldn't stop you acting where it is very obvious. But where decisions which cannot be remade are reached, some level of critical thinking must happen even if this does not progress to a full processing (using hypothetico-deduction).

Figure 3.3 shows a useful way of adopting a method of thinking critically in high-pressure situations requiring action. Take a moment to walk through the flowchart using different scenarios you have faced in practice and see which route you take. The first junction in the flowchart, which assesses how typical the situation is, is a very useful prompt and allows a rapid use of experience and intuition based on a repeatable process which takes almost no time at all.

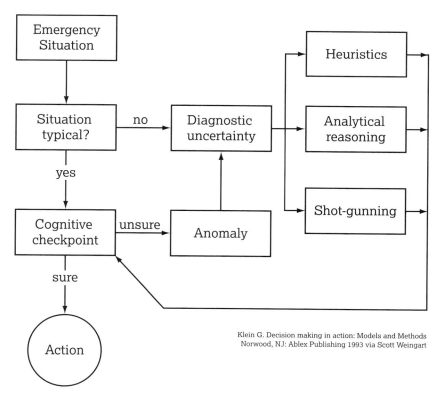

Klein G. Decision making in action: Models and Methods
Norwood, NJ: Ablex Publishing 1993 via Scott Weingart

Figure 3.3: Decision making in action: models and methods (Klein et al.,1993)

Decision Point Management: Taking Control at Each Stage

There is game you may have heard of called bagatelle. It is similar to pinball in that a small ball is sent up to the top of a runway then falls down towards a series of numbered holes at the bottom. These increase in value from the centre out to the ones at the edge. Between the holes and the top of the runway are pins which are intended to deflect the ball randomly, meaning there is no more skill involved in achieving a higher score than a lower score, whereas the ball is far more likely to land in one of the lower scored holes as the pins tend to move the ball away from the centre line. Unlike pinball, there are no flippers to send the ball back up the runway, and other than the speed at which the ball is sent up to the top of the runway, the player's ability to influence the outcome is minimal. This is a useful way to describe the use of decision point management as an alternative to accepting the influence of random acts. Each pin which can randomly deflect you represents the small decisions you make which make up the overall outcome – such as in a diagnostic process. Decision point management requires each pin to become a considered judgement, and for each level to be navigated as an active process, rather than just letting fate take its course. The correct answer is the result of correctly navigating the multiple forks in the road.

If your game of bagatelle has eighteen rows of pins offset to the pins below, and each column has eight or nine pins (see Figure 3.4), could you recall exactly which pins your ball hit? Were your intentions to get a high score met?

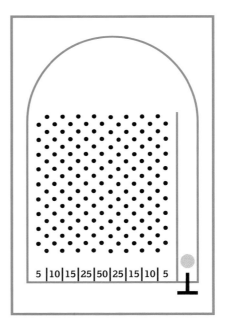

Figure 3.4: Bagatelle 1

While not a decision-making strategy in itself, decision point management is an important tool to use when reviewing and reflecting on the overall outcome, diagnosis or decision. At each point did you know where you were? Did you know the likely outcomes based on each pin hit? Did you think forward as events progressed? Can you look back to see where you should have changed direction? While bagatelle is essentially a random undertaking at the point you launch the ball, by the time it hits the first pin you can start to consider the critical path, albeit in slow time. In much the same way, the level at which an infarct occurs in the coronary circulation and how much collateral circulation the patient has, it is possible to imagine the limitations of which regions of the heart will be affected, and to what degree. In real terms, you can simplify the game by removing pins at each level, localising the possible path for the ball each time it reaches the next level of pins (Figure 3.5).

Once the ball falls between two pins on the top row, the other pins are out of play and so on down the board at each level.

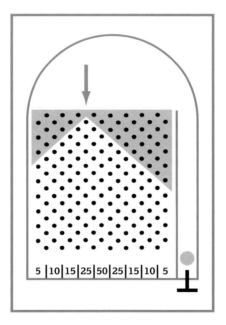

Figure 3.5: *Bagatelle 2*

Figure 3.6 shows the bagatelle board a few levels later. The shaded area is larger still, leaving areas of the playing surface which are unable to be accessed.

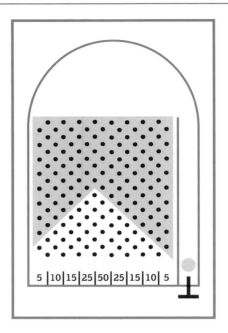

Figure 3.6: *Bagatelle 3*

Figure 3.7 depicts the last level. There are only two possible routes left. In healthcare, these are your final differential diagnoses or impressions. Because you tracked the route through the game, rather than making it random, you can better control the outcome – critically appraising each fork in the road.

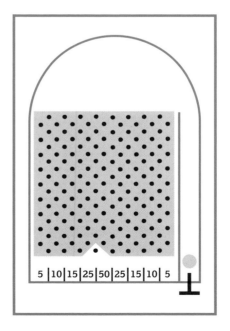

Figure 3.7: *Bagatelle 4*

When thinking critically, imagine where you are on the board and how much of it is irrelevant based on what part of the board cannot be accessed – critically considering what is clearly out of scope (e.g. ignoring pregnancy related issues for male patients). If further down the board you realise that information in another part of the board is needed, you made errors further up the board.

As you get better at critical thinking and have removed the barriers which impede the way to make small conclusions along the way, you will find yourself needing to back-track less. Imagine that the information needed to find the answer to the Humpty Dumpty exercise is higher up the board, and that the critical thinking applied allowed transition through that part of the board. The final piece of the puzzle therefore is entering the board at the correct point to minimise the random nature by which you move down the bagatelle board. Suddenly you have gone from riding the bagatelle board as a passenger, to controlling where the ball enters the game, and can steer each contact with the pins to ensure the route is better controlled. Should you need to go back, you know where the incorrect deviation was made.

Clearly this analogy lacks some of the real-world traits that we see in clinical practice, and the two-dimensional description doesn't lend itself well to the realities of the complex cues, hints and information sources with which we are bombarded. The point about the barriers to critical thinking being ever present and sending you down cognitive blind alleys are illustrated in this method, and as we move ahead you can see how a real-world example is about converting what may feel like a random or self-determining event into a controlled and cognitively derived event. Imagine if the ball represented chest pain as the patient's major symptom group, and instead of scores there were diagnoses across the bottom of the board. How comfortable would you be allowing the diagnosis of indigestion to be made?

Summing Up: Moving from 'What' to 'Why'

The first step towards a hypothetico-deductive decision-making acumen relies on clean data; information which has been filtered and verified before use as a preparatory stage in the decision-making process. It isn't enough to simply say what you see, and being able to satisfy yourself why something is the way it is will assist greatly when higher level decisions are made, and this in turn will ensure your patients are as safe as possible, and allow you to consolidate each experience you have without needing to accept each individual episode as foregone. It is true that with the vast majority of encounters with patients and their pathologies, it will be blindingly obvious what is wrong, but these situations always have a backstory, and it is the acceptance, or otherwise, of what you see that will help you grow as a decision maker and a critical thinker. Establishing the balance between System 1 and System 2 thinking in the context of critical thinking is hard to achieve, and your reliance on each system will develop over time.

By way of example, experienced clinicians may commence cardiopulmonary resuscitation without taking a pulse. At this point the 'what' is unequivocal and becomes paramount with action required immediately (System 1 processing). This instant access to the 'essence of pulselessness' is identical conceptually to the 'essence of cat' in that the context, situation, signs, features and other subtle indications collectively and subconsciously contribute to the correct answer. If you are wrong, the patient will wake up and tell you to get off, and you can then consider the 'why'– why did I initially think they needed CPR? If you are right, you can start asking why they are pulseless in parallel to the essential treatment (System 2 processing).

Conclusion

This chapter has introduced the concept of critical thinking, applied in a practical format intended to promote its use in a way that improves one's approach to that which may appear obvious but may not be correct. It is important to make sure that each situation is approached in such a way that the rapidly emerging picture, based on a wide variety of information, is seen through sceptical and cynical eyes. This will produce the required impetus to be inquisitive and probing. As with many theories and models, the world is rarely that simple, and there will always be other dilemmas and conundrums which need to be overcome in practice.

The next chapter will start to look at the more holistic aspects of decision making, moving the theory into a more parallel position alongside patient-centred care. By the end of the book, the skills discussed will always be subordinate to the patients' needs, rather than being a superficial skill from which the clinician derives satisfaction. Rather, it is the effect this ability has on the patient outcome overall which becomes most important. As you introduce critical thinking into your practice as part of your developing decision-making skills, you will need to start thinking about the other considerations to hone your art, such as improving your communication skills, ethical considerations, managing changing and dynamic environments, and considering the evidence base in the context of patients' needs and wishes.

Reflective Exercises

- Thinking back to the Tenerife Air Disaster example in this chapter, p.38, consider a time when you have worked with a more senior clinician, or have been in a situation where you have witnessed a senior/subordinate team dynamic. What risks were present? Could harm have been caused to the patient? And what techniques could you use to prevent errors caused by this type of issue in the practice setting?

- Consider the list of issues from the section on 'Barriers to Critical Thinking', pp.35–40. Work through the list and note down times where you have been affected by these barriers and consider ways you might control this in the future.

- Think of a time where your decision making felt like a game of bagatelle, and your diagnosis was arrived at without structure and without being able to track back to the start.

Further Resources

Visit www.criticalthinking.org to learn more about critical thinking.

4 Decision Making Theory: Human Factors, Dilemmas and Conundrums

Chapter Objectives

This chapter will cover:

- Defining autonomy;
- Human factors;
- Checklists and structured communication;
- Human fallibility and biased thinking – learn before you make mistakes.

'If you can't explain it simply, you don't understand it well enough.'

'Insanity: doing the same thing over and over again and expecting different results.'

'Everything should be made as simple as possible, but not simpler.'

(Albert Einstein, 1879–1955)

Introduction

Decision making is, by and large, a practised skill. As with any such skill, practice is undertaken to resolve the issues which inhibit proficiency. Expertise is thought to take 10,000 hours cumulatively to achieve, and requires focus on technique and learning to avoid distractions (Syed, 2011). In decision making there are lots of distractions which can affect the development of your improving acumen. This chapter covers some of the issues, many of which may be hidden in plain sight, but understanding more about them can minimise their impact on patient care.

It is important to remember that the human brain is quite new to life in the modern world, and we often hear about the 'old part' and 'new part' of our brains. The studies undertaken by Daniel Kahneman (2011) on heuristics and biases, which won him a Nobel prize, talk of two 'systems' linked to these parts of our minds – System 1 and System 2. System 1 is fast, subconscious, instinctive, and allows us to make rapid decisions based on what is programmed in, based on experience (heuristics). System 2 is slow, deliberate, considered, and is hopeless if you are wondering what to do when being chased by a predator. System 2 is therefore more connected to us as a person, and because we sometimes lack insight into the biases that can fool us into thinking something is correct and logical, but which may be wrong because we allowed ourself to be fooled because of the very fallibilities associated with being human.

The first topic covered in this chapter is autonomy which, while not necessarily a distraction or bias, it is not always well understood in professional practice. Paramedics need to consider the utility of autonomy, as the upholding or preserving of it may become a significant distraction.

Before we move on into the chapter itself, please watch the following film (either type the link below into your browser, or Google 'Monkey Business Illusion') to undertake a quick test of your ability to concentrate on a task which really tests your System 2 mind and your susceptibility to distractions.

- Web Link: https://www.youtube.com/watch?v=IGQmdoK_ZfY
- Google: 'Monkey Business Illusion'

(Simons, 2010)

Defining Autonomy

Healthcare practice has in some ways developed a currency around the term 'autonomy'. When one reflects on its utility, it can be argued that its meaning may be becoming outmoded in the context of modern leadership/followership models. Autonomy could be seen to promote steep hierarchies, create silos, develop barriers and, most importantly, diminish what is important in care: that care of the patient is paramount. If the last chapter resonated with you, perhaps the first concept you would critically appraise is your autonomy; how do you consider autonomy in the context of your practice, your career, and your patients?

So, what is wrong with autonomy? The most basic definition breaks down the Greek origins of the word into 'Autos' meaning self, and 'Nomos' meaning law – suggesting a freedom from external influence and law. It could be argued that laws are rules, and that we are moving away from rule-based practice. But are we? We must reflect on the 'laws' that define our practice, looking at tenets such as evidence-based medicine, clinical governance, peer review and continuing professional development, to name but a few. Perhaps therefore it is better to focus on the use of autonomy in its most positive light: freedom to think and freedom to act but within clear boundaries, which serve to promote patient safety and optimal outcomes.

How many of us consider career progression, or the completion of a course, with the prospect that it will make us 'more autonomous'? Do we really understand what this means for our patients? We don't need to actively celebrate or promote our autonomy as we are all autonomous as human beings. But we do need to understand what this means for our practice and for our patients in relation to decision making. For example, if a paramedic is claiming an enhanced level of autonomy by dint of being an advanced paramedic, does this positively imply unconditional trust in their ability? Or does it negatively suggest professional isolation, elitism and unquestionable authority?

It may seem oxymoronic to suggest practising within a model of 'bounded autonomy' and so autonomy may be inappropriate to emphasise in healthcare practice. Instead perhaps we should look at autonomy in terms of its intrinsic benefits rather than its extrinsic limitations. If we practise effective clinical leadership and followership, we see less of a need to be autonomous and more need to be integrated, trusted, involved and engaged. Autonomy may also imply a pressure to perform in a certain way or act according to a certain expectation, and this is certainly true in paramedic practice – particularly in the ambulance service.

Human Factors

Before starting this section, which is a very brief overview of human factors, I would like to share a specific example of a human factor in practice. The story below describes a personal experience – a meeting with someone who is an expert in human factors and has contributed hugely to patient safety based on his own tragic experiences. This example presents an opportunity to introduce the individual in question and highlight a natural bias in human thought.

Coincidences are a regular reminder of how human beings can delude themselves into thinking that higher powers are at play, or that the presence or proximity of two seemingly random events are uncanny, when in fact it is just the inevitable juxtaposition of the unlikely and unpredictable intersecting. Understanding how human factors affect decision making in healthcare is vital and is a key aspect in preventing avoidable harm, and coincidence is linked to associative bias which can hinder good decision process and outcomes.

Some time ago, I attended a Human Factors Workshop at my local District General Hospital, organised by a fantastic Emergency Department Consultant with a passion for human factors. Hearing about the theory of human factors in practice made the day relevant and highly enjoyable. During the morning, we were shown the video of Martin Bromiley, an airline pilot who lost his wife due to errors made during the induction of anaesthetic for a minor operation, and who went on to share the advances made in the aviation industry with the healthcare sector. Seeing the impact of medical errors as told by the patient's family opened up my eyes to the importance of understanding how we as humans are vulnerable to making avoidable errors. That evening I Googled Martin Bromiley and read more about his experiences. I realised that this man's courage in the face of tragedy, and his resolve to prevent future deaths, is highly inspirational, as his work highlights clearly the fallible nature of human psychology. Martin and his story became etched in my mind.

Two weeks later I found myself taking my seat on a plane at Frankfurt Airport, returning from a conference. I heard the captain announce himself as 'Martin Bromiley'. I cannot tell you the name of the first officer as I was too busy thinking what a coincidence it was that I was being flown by someone that I had only recently been made aware of. At this point, I did what modern humans do in this situation – I tweeted it. A few days later, while reading more about human factors for this book I thought to myself, 'hang on, was this a coincidence?' The fact is if you fly with the airline that a particular pilot is employed by, and you take the route that that pilot regularly works, the chances of being on the same plane is almost routine, and certainly predictable. Moreover, the proximity of that pilot to the reference of human factors is also unremarkable as he is the only pilot so closely linked to human factors in healthcare and so it's not surprising I had heard of him.

In exploring this particular human factor a little more, the presence of coincidences appears more often than we think in everyday life. I wonder how we consider them in clinical practice as, in the context of care, nothing can be considered pre-ordained and probability has less relevance in the final consideration of a patient's condition. This is especially the case when other biases are at play, and when we consider the roles of chance and luck associated with poor decision making and the influence of human factors. Looking back at my experience, we can consider four possible scenarios relating to the example given, from which we can reflect on the likelihood/probabilities. Let's consider the main combinations:

- Being on a plane operated by the same airline that Martin Bromiley flies for, the pilot not being Martin Bromiley, and not knowing who Martin Bromiley is.

- Being on a plane operated by the same airline that Martin Bromiley flies for and the pilot being Martin Bromiley, and not knowing who Martin Bromiley is.

- Being on a plane operated by the same airline that Martin Bromiley flies for and the pilot not being Martin Bromiley, and knowing who Martin Bromiley is.

- Being on a plane operated by the same airline that Martin Bromiley flies for and the pilot being Martin Bromiley, and knowing who Martin Bromiley is.

We can discount 1 and 2 because I know who he is, and therefore 3 is the most likely scenario for me. I actually experienced number 4, which in fact has nothing whatsoever to do with seeing a presentation on human factors with him in it a few weeks before, and comes down simply to mathematical probability. What is more important is that there is a statistical chance of anyone being flown by Martin Bromiley, and this chance is the same whether you are aware of him or not. The important point to note is that a decision made about patient care should never be seen as a coincidence. An understanding of chance and probability must be made, and any hindsight afforded by the outcome should be disregarded in light of previous episodes.

Before moving into human factors more generally, I recommend improving your chances of enjoying the same likelihood of this experience by finding out who Martin Bromiley is by watching the short film called 'Just a Routine Operation'. The content of the film will hopefully give you greater insight into the work done to prevent errors in healthcare, and make you strive for greater understanding of what factors create error, and to consider more the importance of humility when things go wrong. You can find the film by typing this link into your browser, or by searching in Google for '*Just a Routine Operation*'

- Web Link: https://www.youtube.com/watch?v=JzlvgtPIof4

- Google: '*Just a Routine Operation*'

Human factors is a huge topic, and its inclusion in this chapter is only intended as a very high-level view which can lead on to further reading. I have included a short bibliography at the end of this section containing a few books which are essential reading.

Definition of Human Factors

Human factors are, in simple terms, the things that are part of the human condition and which may adversely affect what we do. They highlight the fallibilities which we all have and help to provide ways of gaining an understanding of how these factors can be controlled, and their effects minimised. Human factors demonstrate that human beings did not evolve to be paramedics. From an evolutionary perspective, the human brain is still far more tuned to not being trodden on by a woolly mammoth or being mauled by a sabre-toothed tiger than it is to differentiating the causes of abdominal pain in a patient lying in a pub toilet.

There is an NHS definition of human factors published in 2010:

> '*Enhancing clinical performance through an understanding of the effects of teamwork, tasks, equipment, workspace, culture, organisation on human behaviour and abilities, and application of that knowledge in clinical settings.*'
> (Clinical Human Factors Group, 2015)

Human factors can be divided into the factors which can directly influence individuals and the factors within systems and organisations which can influence individuals and teams. Another important part of human factors is how they change decisions and outcomes. and how these can change decisions and outcomes. Understanding each facet of these factors can assist you when making decisions about a patient's care. Being able to recognise the factors which can negatively influence outcomes which may prevent harm will help make care safer, and your decisions more defensible. The following selection of human factors is taken from the Clinical Human Factors Group, of which Martin Bromiley is a member, and the full list can be downloaded here: http://chfg.org/what-are-clinical-human-factors (CHFG, 2015). Each heading and sub-heading links to explanations of the types of problems that can be experienced in relation to the title. The ones highlighted purple and in **bold** are of particular relevance to paramedic practice and decision making due to the uncertain nature of clinical encounters and the unpredictable environments paramedics practise in.

You may notice that some of these terms are in the glossary and may also be cited in other chapters and sections. This highlights how broad human factors can be, and how significant its impact can be due to it arising in so many areas of practice – and life in general. Some of the factors in Table 4.1 below are negative, but some are positive and provide mitigation.

Heading	Sub-heading	Factor	Example
Organisation	System	Function allocations	Roles at the patients' side, such as in the ambulance setting where a crew allocates 'driver' and 'attendant' roles. This may lead to a loss of control by the lead clinician.
		Functions	Perhaps working in a setting which is under significant pressure, leading to a situation where staff are working functionally in excess of their ability.
		Systems	High levels of demand, absenteeism, resource availability, system design, computer systems and rostering can all lead to system-led human factor issues. Systems may also include policies, procedures, protocols and guidelines.
		Tasks	Tasks must be suitable for the person undertaking them, such as discharging a patient from care.

Heading	Sub-heading	Factor	Example
		Workload	Levels of demand, and work intensity are human factors commonly experienced in healthcare and are cited commonly as contributory factors to error and harm.
	Training	Simulation	The use of simulation is a key method for addressing human factors, rather than being a human factor in its own right. Developing ways to test teams and systems, particularly using high-fidelity models and systems, is proven to reduce the impact of human factors. In aviation, most commercial pilots will never experience a real engine fire, but will undergo high-pressure simulation each year to ensure that the anticipated reactions can be managed.
		Skills gap	Underinvestment in systems and organisations, particularly where funding becomes scarce, can lead to skills gaps. Systems should assess and address any deficiencies in the skills of their workforce in order to mitigate the inherent issues which are associated with sub-optimal ability.
		Training	Inconsistent curricula and methods of teaching, including supervision and mentorship, can be a significant human factor in paramedic practice. Access to primary and refresher training may also be challenging to access – particularly as

Heading	Sub-heading	Factor	Example
		Training *(continued)*	systems get busier and funding becomes ever more scarce.
	Workforce	Competence	The individual clinicians who comprise the workforce must be competent, and many reports (such as inquests) conclude a basic lack of competence to undertake the procedure or intervention which went wrong. Competency should be evidential and subject to robust testing in order to be fully fit for purpose.
		Job design	The roles undertaken by any worker must be well conceived and describe accurately what they are expecting to achieve. It is not uncommon to see roles experience 'scope creep' – a term more commonly used in project management, but aptly describes how a role can deviate from its original purpose, and how this can impact on the intended end-goal. In health, this can mean patient safety and outcomes, as well as clinician wellbeing.
		Personnel and staffing levels	Being part of a system, and being organised into teams and departments is a vital aspect of successful team dynamics, and yet in healthcare we vary teams routinely. One emergency department consultant recently calculated that in his ED there were a possible 16 million permutations of

Heading	Sub-heading	Factor	Example
		Personnel and staffing levels *(continued)*	teams, and yet a Formula 1 pit-crew never varies. Variation often occurs where poor and temporary staffing is used. Clinicians should be wary of periods in practice where the team is new and/or unrehearsed.
		Cognition and **cognitive tasks**	The overarching ability to process information cognitively is a fundamental human factor, as it is so vulnerable to being diminished through factors such as fatigue and hunger.
		Decision making	Decision making is considered a human factor in its own right, and this book's focus on decision making reflects its vital nature in terms of awareness, and the effects of poor decision making.
		Heuristics	Heuristics are the pieces of information for which little or no additional processing is needed and is almost seen as a reflex. Many heuristically driven actions are very useful and link closely to the System 1 part of the brain (reacting to danger or employing psychomotor reactions). Anything that requires deduction, but which is considered as a heuristic skill, could be seen as intuition and be reflected upon.
		Information processing	See section in Chapter 6.

Heading	Sub-heading	Factor	Example
		Memory	We may believe that we have retained everything we have learned and committed them to memory, but how many of us can remember things not in common use? If you work in critical care, could you still recall the names of the muscles in the rotator cuff? Memory is highly fallible and our brain sometimes misleads us. Many crime investigations have demonstrated witnesses providing a testimony based on what they remembered, but which is contradicted by CCTV footage.
		Situational awareness	One of the key strengths of the paramedic profession is strong situational awareness. One only has to consider times when another clinician is undertaking an observer shift on an ambulance to see the impact of a lack of situational awareness. For example, forgetting the situation you are in when attending a road accident may lead to being struck by a vehicle.
		Vigilance	In recent times, the Security Services have reminded travellers on public transport to be vigilant to the threat of terrorism; most commonly by asking the public to be on the lookout for suspicious packages on railway station concourses and other places. This request for vigilance requires a focus on the consequence of a threat, and

Heading	Sub-heading	Factor	Example
		Vigilance *(continued)*	in healthcare this threat is missing something which affects the patient negatively. Red flags are an essential list of signs, symptoms and/or considerations which the clinician must be vigilant towards to minimise risk to the patient and promote good outcomes.
Individual	Team	Communication	Communication within a team is vital, and is often overlooked. How often have we 'heard' but haven't 'listened'? You can test yourself and your colleagues by challenging each other to repeat back any requests given. For instance, when you ask a colleague to go and call for a porter, and on the way back fetch a 500ml bag of saline, ask them what you asked for. It might seem odd to start with, but once embedded it will improve communication.
		Culture, leadership, followership and team behaviours (teamwork)	Leadership and the principles of strong leadership are well established terms in healthcare teams, but good leadership must be complemented by good followership as part of effective team behaviours. Followership doesn't infer loss of autonomy or blind devotion or obedience, rather it demonstrates effective team dynamics.
		Non-technical skills	Many non-technical skills in healthcare have a significant impact on patients. For

Heading	Sub-heading	Factor	Example
		Non-technical skills *(continued)*	example, lifting and handling of patients is essentially a non-technical skill, but where there is a lack of understanding, and where the team doesn't operate effectively, the patient could be harmed. Using a Formula 1 example again, the pit-crew is made up of highly skilled mechanics who have secondary roles during the race. One of the key roles is simply to hold a sign in front of the driver to say when it's safe to leave the pit-box area. The 'Lollipop Man', as the role is known, has little technical skill, but is critical to the entire pit-stop. If he releases a car into the path of another, the team can be penalised and a fatality could happen.
		Shared mental model	The way by which teams operate with a common understanding and purpose. In healthcare, the evidence is still emerging regarding the adoption of this system and may still be considered vague by some.
	Safety	Active errors	These are the kinds of errors with an immediate negative impact or consequence and where the outcome was not intended. An example is where an allergy fails to be taken in to consideration when administering a drug.
		Adverse event	Adverse events are well understood in healthcare, and are defined within key NHS documents. Levels of

Heading	Sub-heading	Factor	Example
		Adverse event *(continued)*	harm suffered by patients are stratified, and 'never events' are closely scrutinised and reported. Many adverse events are minimally harmful, but where they are repeated over and over they become problematic, particularly where these are considered 'near misses' (see Near miss, below).
		Confirmation bias	See the section later in this chapter on Human fallibility and biased thinking
		Human error	Human error refers to any issue or error attributable to the judgement of a human being, rather than a systematic or other failure. In reality, these are quite rare as there is often a system-mediated problem which led to the error. Many aviation accidents were put down to human error in previous eras, whereas modern aviation seeks to identify a root-cause which leads the pilot to make better decisions. The following phrase is apt in relation to human error; 'if you want to encourage something, make it easy. If you want to discourage it, make it hard'.
		Lapses and slips	A lapse may be seen as something that would otherwise not have occurred. A surgeon who has undertaken the same procedure hundreds of times and who once fails to complete a vital intervention may be deemed to have

Heading	Sub-heading	Factor	Example
		Lapses and slips *(continued)*	suffered a lapse – either in concentration, judgement or skill. Healthcare regulators look at lapses and omissions when undertaking Fitness to Practice hearings, and consider the risk of reoccurrence in their judgements.
		Latent error	This is where the error made does not become apparent immediately, and could involve longer term effects from incorrectly prescribed medicines, but it could also involve decisions about ongoing care such as discharging a patient with an incorrect diagnosis leading to deterioration in due course.
		Near miss	Near misses are highly significant events as they indicate a potentially failing system. For example, where staff repeatedly report almost giving the wrong medicine to a patient because it is very similarly packaged, this can be analysed and revisions made to the system in response – for example, repackaging or moving the offending medicine to a different place. In the early 1990s there was a series of errors involving the mistaken contamination of saline flushes with potassium vials, leading to patients receiving fatal doses instead of isotonic and harmless sodium chloride. There were countless near misses leading

Heading	Sub-heading	Factor	Example
		Near miss *(continued)*	up to the first fatal error. This highlights the importance of reporting with confidence, and the maintenance of a safety culture (see below).
		Omissions	This is what it says on the tin – omitting a key aspect of care or other intervention essential to patient care. For example, forgetting to administer prophylactic antibiotics after an operation without good reason may be considered an omission.
		Redundancy	Another positive response to human factors is redundancy. This is where a back-up, or a parallel process is built into systems which promotes continuity in the event of a breakdown or error (for example, aircraft have multiple hydraulic systems rather than rely on only one). In more human focused activity, using a scribe or reading a checklist provides redundancy to the fallible human memory should an individual forget something.
		Resilience	Resilient systems are responsive to demands and are designed to operate consistently regardless of fluctuations – such as demand levels. If a rise in demand leads to more short-term staff absenteeism, the system is not sufficiently resilient.

Heading	Sub-heading	Factor	Example
		Safety culture	This is a vital trait of a successful system. Healthcare settings which have a safety culture embrace error and report freely and confidently. Safety culture requires staff to feel confident to speak up, and aims to learn from all incidents and near misses.
		System safety	The way that the entire system is designed end-to-end to ensure safety in a joined up, cohesive way, and which reduces risk to users.
	Contributory Factors	Distractions and interruptions	In paramedic practice, as with most aspects of healthcare practice, there are lots of opportunities to become distracted during interventions, which can lead to error. Some areas of healthcare have developed processes to remove distraction, but this is not always possible in all circumstances.
		Fatigue	This is a common issue for all healthcare workers, and in recent times, paramedics in particular. The impact of fatigue – either through lack of sleep, rotating shifts, or work intensity – has significant impact on a person's ability to concentrate and undertake cognitive tasks. Seeking support where fatigue is felt is a key feature of professional insight and patient safety.

Heading	Sub-heading	Factor	Example
		Stress	This is best taken verbatim from the CHFG document: 'The physical, mental and emotional response in reaction to demands placed upon people. Some stress can improve performance, excessive stress leads to deterioration in performance.' (CHFG, 2015, p.20)
	User Centred Design	**Anthropometrics**	How appropriate equipment is designed and used in relation to user comfort. For example, being able to raise and lower an ambulance stretcher reduces physical stress and risk of injury to staff and patients.
		Devices	Healthcare practice uses a vast array of devices to diagnose, monitor and treat patients. Devices should be fit for purpose and used according to their design. Modification or adaptation of devices can lead to a risk of harm for patients and staff.
		Ergonomics	Taken verbatim from the CHFG document: 'Understanding the skills and abilities of paramedics, i.e. users, and their emergency care tasks, informs the design of new ambulances and of mobile treatment units.' (CHFG, 2015, p.10)
		Human system interface	The interaction between humans in a designed system. For example, making a referral via a pre-existing care pathway.

Heading	Sub-heading	Factor	Example
		Link analysis	Determining the space needed for a task to be carried out in the working environment. This can be analysed dynamically, such as when considering carrying out an intervention while the patient is *in situ* (e.g. stuck in a small space) or after moving them to a better working space.
		Packaging, labelling and signage	Medicines errors can occur where vials appear very similar and/or if unfamiliar doses of the same medicine are introduced into a clinical setting leading to under/overdose.
		Physical environment	The influence the work environment has on performance. For example, carrying out a resuscitation in a hot and noisy nightclub may be more challenging than in a resuscitation room in an emergency department.
		Target audience description	The description and/or attributes of the person intended to use a particular system or piece of equipment. For instance, Hazardous Area Response Team (HART) members using specialist off-road vehicles.
		Usability	How easily a system or piece of equipment can be used. Systems or processes which are clunky or convoluted are often not adhered to, or workarounds are adopted. If a system isn't usable, it may be unsafe.

Heading	Sub-heading	Factor	Example
		User centred design	Using users and recipients of systems and services to assist in the design to ensure usability and suitability.
		Workplace design	Ensuring that the workspace is fit for purpose.

Table 4.1: Selection of Human Factors (Clinical Human Factor Group, 2015)

Activity

Download and read the PDF of this guide from the Clinical Human Factors Group and take some time to consider these problems and solutions in the context of your organisation, colleagues and patients. Think about how the tools and techniques could be used to make improvements. How could you change what you do in order to minimise any negative effects of your practice and work environment? How would you raise any concerns you have about these issues in your organisation?

- Web Link: http://www.chfg.org/how-to-guide-to-human-factors-volume-1/
- Google: 'Clinical Human Factors Group'

Table 4.2 shows an example of one of these headings, taken from the Clinical Human Factors Group document on staffing levels.

Staffing levels	Having the right people in the right place at the right time. Ensuring that they have suitable knowledge, skill and experience to operate safely.	The number of staff, task demands and shift lengths that are balanced to deal with the unexpected workload, e.g. the ratio and skill mix of registered nurses and healthcare assistants on a ward.	Having the right staff in a supermarket based on the likely number of customers at both quiet and busy times, staff trained to work at the checkout, stack shelves, make deliveries or manage the store.

Table 4.2: Safe staffing levels (Clinical Human Factors Group, 2015)

There are methods of systematically preventing errors arising from the influence of human factors. The full list is also available in the Clinical Human Factors Group document and includes two vitally important processes which are highly relevant in paramedic practice, but are not exploited to the full – checklists and structured communication.

Checklists and Structured Communication

The Clinical Human Factors Group (2015) defines a checklist as: '*A job aid designed to concisely summarise the key elements of a task as an aid to memory and ensure correct procedures are followed.*'

It is entirely unrealistic for human beings to retain the volume of information associated with professional practice, and yet we commonly see omissions attributed to 'human error'. These can be more specifically assessed as relating to the challenges humans face in day-to-day life. We must recognise this if we want to embrace a learning culture. The term '**no blame culture**' is more commonly referred to, but 'learning culture' better describes how issues must be kept on the radar rather than given to someone or something under the banner of blame.

Were we to replace our human professional workforce with automatons, we wouldn't need to worry about the limitations associated with humans – fatigue, stress, hunger, personal problems, shift working, illness, etc. as machines don't get tired or hungry, they are not moved by emotional experiences, they don't have arguments with their partners or have any stress. They could store all the information they would ever need in an infinitely expandable hard-drive and be able to recall expertly every disease and treatment, regardless of how infrequently they presented. The problem of course is that the patient would receive little or no care or compassion – core tenets of healthcare (NHS England, 2014a). So we tolerate the limitations of humans because the essence of healthcare relies on higher concepts such as empathy. The next best thing to trying to create a caring robot is to help humans behave in a more robot-like way at times where recall may be affected by extrinsic factors. This is where checklists come in.

Checklists have existed in the airline industry for decades, and every aspect of an aircraft's flight is covered by a checklist: *before-start, after-start, before take-off, after take-off/climb, approach, landing, after-landing, parking* – to name but a few. Each of the checklists serve to remove variations from the process and remove the risk of omission – a very simple principle, but one which has not had the same level of adoption in healthcare, except for a few very notable examples, such as the WHO Surgical Checklist (WHO, 2008) which has reduced surgical errors by around 50%.

One area of paramedic practice which has fully embraced the use of checklists is critical care (HEMS and Specialist/Advanced Paramedics in Critical Care) where high-risk interventions are undertaken using detailed checklists to prepare equipment, identify roles and responsibilities, what drugs are being given and, very importantly, what the contingencies are should things go wrong. The checklist process also introduces more clear and structured communication, setting up the team in such a way that minimises risks of miscommunication.

Checklists have four main types (static parallel, static sequential with verification, static sequential with verification and confirmation, and dynamic) (Winters et al., 2009) but in essence they all work by providing a prompt which requires a response. Checklists can function with a single person, or a whole team, and the level of variation is informed by the level of certainty required.

It is important to consider checklists as a strong ally, and not something which diminishes your professional status. It is not a requirement of practice to remember everything, and the fact is most people cannot go shopping without forgetting something important if they do not have a shopping list. It is unlikely anyone would base their ego and sense of self-worth on the basis of remembering a shopping list, so why would healthcare professionals seek to remember the list of things that need doing – particularly when we consider the hostile and dynamic environments we practise in? Our patients will not be impressed with our powers of recall were we able to remember everything that needs doing. In contrast though, if we fail to recall something vital, the negative effect on them may be huge.

Human Fallibility and Biased Thinking: Learn Before You Make Mistakes

Throughout this chapter, mention has been made of distractions, fallacies, and biases. But what does this actually mean? What we have discussed in regards to Daniel Kahneman's work on the way we as humans think earlier in this chapter touched on the way external influences can be ignored – who saw the gorilla in the YouTube clip, but missed the player leaving and the curtain changing colour? To expand on this, and to ensure that these concepts can be recognised and intercepted when applying a hypothetic-deductive decision-making process, the different influences which can be identified have been expanded with examples of where they can affect patient care. It is worth bearing in mind that Daniel Kahneman is not a healthcare professional, rather he is a psychologist and economist. Many of his examples relate to decision making in economics, and none relate directly to healthcare. There is a good reason why the word 'clinical' has been dropped from 'clinical decision making' – decision making is a human endeavour, and the subject matter which is affected by the decision is process-agnostic. You can misdiagnose a patient, choose the wrong investment portfolio, or buy the wrong size jumper in the clothes store – all based on the same fallibilities associated with the psychology of decision making. With this in mind, decision-making skills are transferrable across all aspects of your life (a rare thing in healthcare), so enjoy.

The next section will look first at Kahneman's main biases which relate most relevantly to clinical practice, after which there is a table which gives examples of other relevant biases and fallacies.

Anchoring

Anchoring is the effect where we tend to allow ourselves to be influenced by numbers which may be irrelevant. While this is most prevalent in consumer psychology – setting a price-point which is acceptable to customers upon which all other prices are set – healthcare has many numbers associated with it, mainly the display of physiological values on monitoring devices and which are contextualised against an anchored normal range.

How often have you looked at a patient who is clearly not unwell, but the pulse oximeter shows a heart rate of 250 bpm and oxygen saturations of 45%? We tend to believe what we see because we anchor a nominal normal for these values, and more usually have a low tolerance for values which appear catastrophic. In this case, a poor signal is almost always the problem and while considering intervention is appropriate, the global picture of the patient leads you to review the quality of the data first.

Consider the 65 kg female involved in a minor collision in their car. 'Normal' blood pressure is 120/80, but this patient's BP is 85/55 – is this abnormal? Is the patient compensating? When you consider the wider picture, and on speaking to the patient (who you are trying to wrestle onto to the trolley in order to raise her legs in the air) she reports that this is her normal blood pressure. If this scenario involved a 200 kg male, the anchoring would be more useful. In this case, though, it's a heuristic bias.

Availability

We tend to err towards that which is available mentally or practically. **Ideation** can be linked to the bias of availability, and can have strange logical outcomes. For example, does working in an ambulance increase the chances of deciding to take a patient to hospital compared to when working on a response car? Does the presence of the availability of transport make the decision easier as it's more available? Clearly, the decision to convey must be based on the patient's needs, and not extrinsic factors.

Also, availability is linked to the consequence of a decision and the perception of its outcome where the thought is close at hand. For example, you are working at an ambulance station where a colleague was recently the subject of an investigation following a complaint about discharging a patient from scene. While the investigation demonstrated no case to answer, the anxiety relating to being investigated increased the number of patients taken to hospital in the period following the investigation, compared to the neighbouring station in the same city. The most available thought was related to consequence, and this in turn affected decisions for patients despite the actual or statistical chance of facing disciplinary action from a complaint (particularly if you make good decisions).

Conjunction Bias

'Conjunction' is simply where events happen at the same time, and where it occurs as a bias it explains where the connection of events can lead to a connection of cause – sometimes incorrectly.

Poorly made intuitive judgements can be highly unethical, and seriously compromise clinical practice, where the **conjunction bias** is present. For example, is it more likely that the incident you are responding to will be perceived negatively if the patient with 'chest pain' is a homeless person than if the patient is living in a detached house in suburbia? This judgement can play out, and the homeless person's needs may not match the initial call. But likewise, the call to the middle-class home may also yield a judgement that it would have been better to see a pharmacist or go to the GP. The important consideration is that if you *must* judge the appropriateness of a 999 call, you should only do it at the end of the incident! Providing subjective information as a series of attributes in a conjoined way, and in an unweighted way, creates a picture which may belie the actual need. The way in which patients enter urgent and emergency care systems makes conjunction more likely, as the information is often truncated and lacks context.

The conjunction bias was discovered through an experiment which Kahneman carried out, called 'The Linda Problem', and provided some very scant information about a made-up subject. Those taking part in the experiment were asked to consider the most likely answer. The research subjects were told that Linda is *'young, single, outspoken, and very bright, who, as a student, was deeply concerned with discrimination and social justice'* (Tversky and Kahneman,1982), and were then asked to decide if Linda was a Bank Teller or a feminist Bank Teller. The question omits the qualifying statements needed to avoid making a decision which in terms of probability is less likely, and the outcome showed the majority of the subjects assumed Linda was a feminist. In terms of probability, the chances of Linda being a Bank Teller is significantly higher than her being a feminist Bank Teller, and the information provided gives no definite suggestion of feminism. The conjunction of the information led to the bias.

The issue relates to what is implied rather than what is correct, avoiding the instinctive answer, and this requires parking all assumptions and social taboos. When making decisions in practice, consider carefully the information you are provided with compared to the information you may seek to elicit. The latter is easier to qualify and can help avoid the conjunction bias.

Optimism and Loss Aversion

In the next chapter, we look at how we approach what we know and what we may not know (**known knowns**, **known unknowns** etc.) and this demonstrates how we tend towards optimism and overconfidence. In practice, clinicians may be inclined towards optimism or pessimism due to their previous experience of a particular disease or patient outcome, and if pessimism develops it may impede good decision making due to the phenomenon of '**loss aversion**'. For instance, this may mean that it is preferred to get every patient with a pulse to hospital regardless of the prognosis rather than 'call it' on scene, as this removes the perceived loss, or guards against unrealistic expectations of the outcome. It could be argued that, in paramedic practice, the balance between optimism and pessimism occurs on a patient-by-patient basis, for example the patient whose injuries are clearly incompatible with life but for whom everything is done to demonstrate absolute futility by evidencing no response to all available interventions, are approached with determination, but ultimately pessimism. Conversely, the patient you hand over at hospital, for whom the long-term outcome is unclear, is left with a feeling of optimism. Either way, the aversion to loss in the healthcare setting is not healthy for the clinician and needs to be understood and recognised, and perhaps for all patients to be approached optimistically, and also realistically (Kahneman, 2011).

There are dozens of biases and fallacies which have been identified in human psychology, many of which are relevant to healthcare decision making. The 2013 book by Rolf Dobelli, presents a list of 100 biases and fallacies. Dobelli collates these into a series of real-world examples which support the title *The Art of Thinking Clearly*. Many of these have direct links to the challenges related to decision making in paramedic practice, and healthcare in general. They are listed in Table 4.3 below with practice examples relevant to patient care.

Bias	Practice Example
Confirmation Bias	The writer Aldous Huxley said that facts do not cease to exist if they are simply ignored, and confirmation bias is where information is omitted or altered to fit a more convenient answer. This is at the heart of good decision making, and is the basis for ensuring good hypotheses are created and tested, and that the unknown unknowns are considered. This bias is always at the top of list as it requires key professional attributes, such as insight and humility, in order to prevent problems. The patient who 'fits' nicely into a diagnosis by omitting the confounding factors is at risk of their clinician being subject to confirmation bias. For example, the 39-year-old male with no family history of cardiovascular disease, and who has a three-day history of fever and productive cough, must be suffering chest pain due to his chest infection. He has been coughing a lot and is too young to be having a heart attack. WRONG – he is *ALSO* having a **myocardial infarction** and will be dead within the next 3 hours.

Bias	Practice Example
Authority Bias	The airline industry, as mentioned at the start of the chapter, has learned much about authority bias in its development of CRM (cockpit resource management), and which has developed in wider settings as 'Crew Resource Management'. The basic premise of CRM is that the most senior person isn't always correct, and the hierarchies can conspire to cause sometimes catastrophic outcomes, as we saw in the example involving Martin Bromiley's wife. One of the key examples of authority bias was the Tenerife air disaster on 27 March 1977 (see Chapter 3). This demonstrated the issue of the relationship between a higher authority who was wrong, and the inability of the junior pilot, whose belief was correct, to challenge the decision. Luckily for paramedics, our practice settings are more and more in tune with CRM. The risk of authority bias still exists and we must be prepared to speak up. For example, the very new HEMS Doctor who wishes to extricate a patient in a certain way that will clearly not work can be approached in a polite and professional way and will be receptive to the challenge. This will mean the patient gets the best care.
Outcome/Hindsight Bias	It is important to judge each decision on the process used rather than the outcome. This links closely to the need to be very cautious if basing your practice entirely upon experience and intuition as the diagnoses, treatment choices and outcomes may merely be a long string of lucky guesses! A good decision may lead to the wrong answer, and a bad decision can lead to the correct answer. Regardless of the outcome, however, a poorly made decision is always the wrong answer. In other words, judge the outcome on how you arrived at the answer rather than the answer itself. Using a decision-making process makes practice as safe as possible and allows the clinician to focus on the patient's episode of care, rather than just whether the outcome is optimised.

Bias	Practice Example
Overconfidence Bias	We all like to think we get things right most of the time, but humans are intrinsically prone to overestimating their ability, and focus on positive experiences when assessing competency.
	In clinical care, forecasting what is wrong with the patient based on the confidence of the clinician is a potentially dangerous way to make complex decisions. **Experiential** and entirely intuitive decision making is covered in subsequent chapters, and the associated concepts which exist alongside overconfidence must be understood by clinicians in order to promote good care for patients. Professional insight and humility are opportunities to promote healthy levels of confidence in practice.
	It is possible that an unbroken run of absence of failure can lead to overconfidence in subsequent encounters; feeding a false sense of security built up over time. This can also link to the authority-biased behaviours where the overconfident clinician demonstrates poor leadership due to the overconfidence in their ability and an unwillingness to be challenged.
	Try this quick exercise. How many diseases could you name that are linked to a chief complaint of abdominal pain? Next, estimate the diagnostic certainty you have when assessing patients with abdominal pain. The literature suggests that diagnoses associated with abdominal pain are wrong 50% of the time, and the list of conditions is upwards of 50. If you named half the conditions, and accept the published diagnostic accuracy, there are little grounds for overconfidence!
Base-Rate Neglect	This bias is linked to 'The Linda Problem' (Tversky and Kahneman,1982) and highlights the issue with failing to appreciate the underlying statistical probabilities of the decisions you make. Consider the following variation on the Linda Problem:
	Chuck is white, lives in Los Angeles and has committed two murders. Is Chuck most likely to be (A) a member of a Hell's Angels motorcycle chapter, or (B) a corporate lawyer?

Bias	Practice Example
Base-Rate Neglect *(continued)*	There are 1.2 million lawyers in the USA, and, according to the US Justice Department, 2500 Hell's Angels worldwide. So while it seems most plausible that Chuck is a Hell's Angels member, it is statistically more likely that he is a lawyer. The intuitive leap to assuming he is a Hell's Angel is an example of base-rate neglect. While good decision making should always take into consideration that rare things happen (rarely), the most likely outcome is most likely. In healthcare, the challenge is to prove that Chuck ISN'T a member of the Hell's Angels, rather than proving he is lawyer. Using abdominal pain again as an example, a 14-year-old male with **right iliac fossa** tenderness is most likely to have appendicitis but could also have an **ischaemic bowel** or a **hernia**. The base-rate instance of appendicitis is far greater than the other two differential diagnoses, both of which must be excluded.
False Causality Bias	A very obvious example of false causality is how low blood glucose can mimic very closely stroke symptoms. A real-world instance of this happened to me in the mid-1990s while I was working as an Ambulance Technician, alongside a paramedic colleague. We were sent to a call for a patient who had been seen at home by the GP who had noted her outward clinical signs: loss of coordination and tone, lack of speech etc., and had called for an ambulance to take the patient to hospital, most likely to die within a few hours due to the severity of the stroke he had diagnosed. The GP left the patient with her family to await our arrival. We were greeted by about 20 family members who all lived close by, and who were all gathering in a highly distressed state, as the GP had told the immediate family about the imminent demise of their mother. We were shown to her bedroom and after a couple of minutes became suspicious about how she was presenting. On doing some simple observations, including blood glucose testing, we found her to be profoundly hypoglycaemic, and reversed this with Glucagon (a medicine which mobilises stores of glucose from the liver). As she began to wake I was tasked by the paramedic to find some oral carbohydrates, and so went down to ask the family if they had any digestive biscuits.

Bias	Practice Example
False Causality Bias *(continued)*	They seemed a little surprised that the ambulance crew were peckish enough to ask for biscuits, and I did fail to provide the full update at that stage.
	Fifteen minutes later, we walked the lady down the stairs into the living room to gasps of shock from the family. We explained what happened, and placed a call to the GP to say what we had done, and would he still like us to take her to hospital, or would he like to return to make a further assessment. He chose to send her in.
	This case highlights the risk of leaping to an obvious conclusion based on false causality. The signs and symptoms suggested stroke, but this was not the correct diagnosis. Stroke, along with hypoglycaemia, should have been a hypothesis (differential diagnosis) at this stage.
Action Bias	'Quick, do something!' Paramedics often hear this when they arrive at an incident, and it can jolt us into 'action bias' – doing something rather than nothing to avoid appearing ineffective. Many actions are very useful to buy time (such as taking a pulse, for instance), but where a decision is made rashly, using only intuition rather than consideration, it may be harmful. Clearly, there are times when immediate action is the only sensible course of action, such as starting CPR where a patient is pulseless, but where these actions can cause further problems, taking time to consider next steps is vital. The tendency towards action bias is often considered in human factors, and the mantra '10 seconds for 10 minutes' is often used to describe how not acting and spending a few seconds sense checking can save so much more time if the alternative is spending 10 minutes undoing the wrong thing.
	In high pressure situations, it takes strong leadership to avoid action bias, and the 10 seconds you spend thinking can feel like a lifetime, but is usually a stitch in time!
Omission Bias	Omission bias may be seen at the opposite of action bias, but it is a little more involved than that. Omission bias is best described by the term often heard in healthcare settings – 'if in doubt, don't'. Arguably, this term is outmoded and may be hard to defend.

Bias	Practice Example
Omission Bias *(continued)*	Consider this scenario: an American paramedic moves to the UK and joins his local ambulance service. It is the early 1990s and he is surprised how few interventions UK paramedics can do compared to the US. A few weeks into his time in the UK he is called to a patient choking in a restaurant. Basic manoeuvres are unsuccessful, and so he begins to consider undertaking a surgical airway, but is reminded that in the UK this is outside his remit. The patient finally goes into cardiac arrest, secondary to the airway occlusion. The fear of consequence leads the paramedic not to act and he continues with basic techniques and conveying the patient to the nearest A&E where a junior doctor carries out an emergency tracheostomy. Sadly, the patient is well beyond help. The hospital complains to the ambulance service asking why someone who is trained was not able to intervene. The ambulance service defends the actions of the paramedic. The coroner cannot provide any comfort to the family in the inquest as the system at the time was biased to omission. There were cases in this period where paramedics acted outside their scope of practice (action bias) with variable outcomes depending on the effect on the patient. Morally it appears hard to justify, and there is no easy answer. Imagine it in these terms: what is the difference between you pushing someone off a cliff and failing to prevent someone falling off a cliff? The outcome is the same – the person dies in the fall – and the influence you have only differs in the physical contact. Consider the difference of patient outcomes in the context of not acting in a dynamic environment, and the potential end result. Not acting may not be any better than acting. A moral and practical dilemma!
Averages Bias	Averages are very useful in retrospect or at the end of a defined period, such as a season's batting average in cricket, average lap times in motorsport, and response times in ambulance services. The problem with averages is that they take time to settle, and can be influenced by large or aberrant data. Many paramedics lament their poor **ROSC** rates compared to colleagues, or their conveyance rates for all

Bias	Practice Example
Averages Bias *(continued)*	their patients – all in short periods of time. Specialist paramedics in urgent care roles may spend all shift dealing with chest pains and serious trauma, sending all their patients to hospital and achieving a 100% conveyance rate that day. Over the course of a year, that one day will be lost very quickly in the averages, and the successful resuscitations will fluctuate for so many reasons, such as **aetiologies**, demography, and geography, to the point where the overall organisational results are unaffected, and all patients receive gold standard care. The risk of averages is the desire to force them – such as taking more risks with patients discharged from the scene in order to reverse a climbing conveyance rate, or ignoring advanced directives and resuscitating patients who are not suitable for resuscitation. A bus carrying 50 people, each earning on average $50,000 dollars per year, is then boarded by Mark Zuckerberg, the founder of Facebook. At this point, the average earning on that bus becomes around $950m. None of the other passengers feel any richer though. The average is so skewed by the spike that it is rendered useless. On a worldwide level, the influence of Zuckerberg's wealth increases the average by only a few dollars, and yet his personal wealth is unchanged. Trying to achieve an average is not always helpful, and many quality improvement systems use statistical process control to give upper and lower control limits based on standard deviations from the mean to give a truer and more meaningful display of performance data, which also provides the opportunity to assess data points that fall outside the upper and lower controls.

Table 4.3: Types of bias

Conclusion

The next chapter looks in detail at hypothetico-deduction as a way of supporting good decision making in practice, and this chapter has looked at the cognitive fogs and biases we all suffer as human beings. Making choices and decisions is for the most part an unconscious process. We do not spend large amounts of time choosing what to wear each day, nor are we particularly aware of when we switch on the car headlamps – we simply reach an intuitive judgement based on the weather or reach a threshold at which point we think the lights should go on. These day-to-day decisions are limited in their consequence (we might spend the day feeling cold, or get flashed by another motorist to warn us our lights aren't on). Many other decisions are more significant and are blighted by the way we interpret the perceived outcome, and this leads to highly illogical but totally understandable behaviours.

The reference materials which have been cited in this chapter are well worth reading in more depth. The least academic, but most entertaining, book is *The Art of Thinking Clearly* by Rolf Dobelli and it seems fitting to leave this chapter with a conundrum based on Dobelli's chapter called 'Would you wear Hitler's Sweater?' which typifies the human condition using the example of contagion bias.

> *You go into a charity shop and find an old sweater in excellent condition in your size. It is clearly very old indeed, and with antique clothing in demand you think this would make an excellent purchase. You go to the checkout and the shopkeeper gives you a very important piece of history about the previous owner of the sweater – it belonged to Adolf Hitler/Jimmy Savile/Ian Brady/Peter Sutcliffe (delete as appropriate). So, would you wear it? No one will know who it belonged to. It's a bargain, it fits, and it's in excellent condition, so why not? Some decisions will always be fogged by biases and these distractions cannot always be avoided. Who would want to walk around in Hitler's cast-offs, regardless of how illogical it would seem, and yet the emotional response it creates means that the illogical decision is probably the one the majority would go with?*
>
> (Based on Dobelli, 2013, pp.166–168)

So, the decision itself may not be the most important aspect of the episode, but navigating your way to the decision certainly is. Thinking back to Chapter 3, can you find your way back to the point where you took each fork in the road? The next chapter opens up a more cyclical and less linear approach, and will start you on a journey to a decision-making acumen.

Reflective Exercises

- Think back to the previous activity on p.68 where you reflected on the list of human factors. Pick one which resonates with you and expand it into a case-based example you have experienced, focusing on the implications for your practice of the factor you selected.

- Pick a bias from the list earlier in the chapter and consider a time where you fell victim to the bias you have chosen. This can be in your personal life or professional life. Remember that consumer psychology relies on these biases, so you may want to consider a scenario outside healthcare, perhaps when you made a purchase.

- Reflect on your autonomy, and your understanding of the term in the context of your professional practice. Consider the human factors relating to team behaviours and safety culture, and how these link to the outcomes for patients.

Human Factors Bibliography

- Clinical Human Factors Group (2015) *Human Factors in Healthcare: Common Terms.* Available: http://chfg.org/what-are-clinical-human-factors. Last accessed July 2016.

- Dobelli, R (2013) *The Art of Thinking Clearly.* London: Spectre.

- Gambrill, E (2012) *Critical Thinking in Clinical Practice*, 3rd ed. Hoboken, USA: John Wiley & Sons Inc.

- Rosenorn-Lanng, D (2014) *Human Factors in Healthcare.* Oxford: Oxford University Press.

- Standing, M (2017) *Clinical Judgement and Decision Making for Nursing Students*, 3rd ed. London: Learning Matters (Sage).

- Winters, B.D., Gurses, A.P., Lehmann, H., Sexton, J.B., Rampersad, C.J. and Pronovost, P.J. (2009) Clinical Review Checklist – translating evidence into practice. *Critical Care*, 13(210): 2.

5 The Garden Path Test: Putting Decision Making into Practice – Intuition, Experience, Hypotheses, and Deduction

Chapter Objectives

This chapter will cover:

- Intuition – how we use this in our everyday life and implications for safe paramedic practice;

- Experience – an exploration of the Benner model 'From Novice to Expert' and Dreyfus's 'Model of Expertise'. We consider how these can be applied in our decision making;

- Hypotheses & Deduction – how to make a clinical decision based on the appropriate evidence and review it.

Introduction

This chapter is called 'The Garden Path Test', and so we had better explain what this is and how a garden path links to decision making. The Garden Path Test is a way of challenging yourself, ensuring that you have confidence in your decisions and that you are confident that you have provided the best care for your patient. The test originated from the experience of getting to the patient's garden gate after leaving them at home following a 999 call, and already worrying whether your decision was correct. If you find yourself reaching for the gate latch and are already considering the consequences if things go wrong, you have made the wrong decision – even if the decision is technically correct! Doubting yourself in this way may mean you have not made an unequivocal and defensible decision, and it's really important for your own wellbeing that you move on from each completed encounter in order to focus on caring for your next patient.

Moving theory into practice can be very challenging, and the dilemmas discussed in the previous chapters all link to the concepts discussed in this chapter. These concepts will lead to new skills which can be used in clinical encounters. As with all skills, once these have been acquired they need to be consolidated to ensure that the approach can be used effectively in patient care. It is vital to promote confidence in clinical practice, and there are plenty of opportunities to create anxiety – particularly if you are making complex decisions.

This chapter will focus on understanding the concepts of experience and intuition and how to approach their use safely and positively in practice. It will also look at how to develop hypotheses and how to test them, and finally how to apply a method of deduction and retesting to find the correct answer. While the focus is mainly on **diagnostic reasoning**, there will be a theme running throughout which suggests ways of also using these concepts in non-diagnostic areas (for instance, building a picture of neglect in a vulnerable person), and with clinical dilemmas where the decision cannot be reached with a definitive diagnosis, or even an impression of the patient's chief complaint. Remember too that the decision to give a medicine is the culmination of a diagnostic process and forms an important aspect of practice.

By the end of this chapter you will have a much better idea of how to approach decision-making dilemmas in everyday practice, and you will begin to develop your decision-making skills by putting theory into practice. This will then take you on into the next chapter which will look in detail at drawing together these separate concepts and linking them into a single process which can improve the way you make decisions and judgements, and which will be safer for your patients and make your role more enjoyable and less stressful.

HCPC Standards

The HCPC makes the following points about ensuring you practise safely and competently:

Taken from Standards of Conduct, Performance & Ethics: http://www.hcpc-uk.org/publications/standards/index.asp?id=38

- *You must act in the best interests of service users.*
- *You must keep high standards of personal conduct.*
- *You must keep your professional knowledge and skills up to date.*
- *You must act within the limits of your knowledge, skills and experience and, if necessary, refer the matter to another practitioner.*
- *You must communicate properly and effectively with service users and other practitioners.*

If you make informed, reasonable and professional judgements about your practice, with the best interests of your service users as your prime concern, and you can justify your decisions if you are asked to, it is very unlikely that you will not meet our standards.

By 'informed', we mean that you have enough information to make a decision. This would include reading these standards and taking account of any other relevant guidance or laws. By 'reasonable', we mean that you need to make sensible, practical decisions about your practice, taking account of all relevant

*information and the best interests of the people who use or are affected by your
services. You should also be able to justify your decisions if you are asked to.*

(HCPC, 2016)

Taken from Standards of Proficiency: http://www.hcpc-
uk.org/publications/standards/index.asp?id=48

Registrant paramedics must:

- be able to practise as an autonomous professional, exercising their own professional judgement.

- be able to assess a professional situation, determine the nature and severity of the problem and call upon the required knowledge and experience to deal with the problem.

- be able to make reasoned decisions to initiate, continue, modify or cease treatment or the use of techniques or procedures, and record the decisions and reasoning appropriately.

- recognise that they are personally responsible for and must be able to justify their decisions.

- be able to make a decision about the most appropriate care pathway for a patient and refer patients appropriately.

- **understand the following aspects of clinical science:**

  - the theoretical basis of assessment, clinical decision making and appropriate treatment plans, along with the scientific evaluation of their effectiveness

  - the theories supporting problem solving and clinical reasoning

(HCPC, 2014)

Intuition – The Enemy Within?

This section explores intuition, along with both the benefits and the dangers to which it can give rise. In particular, the chapter urges caution about using intuition alone, without searching for facts to confirm or counterbalance it.

Intuition can be useful in many areas of life, and implies deep/tacit understanding or expertise. Intuition is driven by imprinted and practised ability (heuristics, and the use of your brain's 'System 1') which is applied most effectively in repetitive tasks requiring high levels of skill. Observe how a racing driver's lap times improve on a track that is gradually drying following a rain shower. The driver knows intuitively how far it is possible to push the car by considering a range of cues, such as what can be observed visually as well as through haptic feedback (what can be felt through the steering wheel). The ability to drive a racing car is learned and practised, but correcting a small skid in dynamic conditions requires instinct and intuition – and these may make the difference between being in pole position and crashing off the track. This suggests that intuition is a largely unconscious process, so it's very important to understand better what intuition is.

The Cambridge Dictionary defines intuition as:

> *'(knowledge from) an ability to understand or know something immediately based on your feelings rather than facts'*
>
> (Cambridge Dictionary, 2017)

And Patricia Benner (1984) describes intuition as *'The rapid grasp of a problem'*.

Why do we allow ourselves to use intuition in clinical practice when the definitions are essentially saying *'you probably get the problem on some level, but you don't need to understand it'*? This sounds somewhat risky! There are of course situations in life where intuition protects us – as in the case of the racing driver we met earlier – and in fact the origin of intuition itself comes from the oldest parts of the human brain which prevented us from being eaten by large, unfriendly creatures. This therefore reminds us that intuition requires no mental effort or active cognitive load. Our prehistoric forebears did not stand on the savannah debating with each other about whether or not the presence of a sabre-toothed tiger running towards them represented a threat to their personal safety, and if it did what were their range of options? No, they ran the other way and climbed a tree. Instinctively their brain said to them that this animal has large sharp teeth and is also intuitively driven to kill and eat, and to act accordingly. Most importantly, intuition only deals with *'what'* and doesn't require you to ask *'why'*. This is a serious problem in the context of decision making in clinical practice.

In the modern paradigm, there are some situations where intuition provides protection where an immediate and dynamic response is needed, such as swerving to avoid a hazard when driving. This is equivalent to the old part (system 1) of our brain screaming at us as if a sabre-toothed tiger was approaching. Arguably, there are few situations in a clinical encounter at the patient's side that call for such extreme responses. Even diagnosing cardiac arrest and rapidly beginning CPR is not an intuitive response. You may think it is – after all, your intuition tells you the patient is very sick indeed. But this assessment does not imply understanding at anything other than a peripheral level (another example of the need to ask *'why'*). Even when you are so experienced that you probably don't even need to take a pulse in some of your obviously pulseless patients, you still do so to assure yourself that CPR is the right approach. This also gives you the prompt to ask yourself what has caused the condition (and how you might reverse it – *why* is this patient in cardiac arrest). These unconsciously stored items of knowledge, and their rapid or automatic recall, are known as heuristics, and there is a specific example of heuristic behaviour known as **affect heuristics**, where one-dimensional cues create a response. A common example of this is how words are received and responded to. Hearing the phrase 'terrorist attack' creates a negative reaction, whereas 'lottery win' creates a positive one. It is important to challenge yourself and to ensure that you ask *why*, as heuristics will only give you the *what*.

In less immediate circumstances, time is your friend and intuition is your enemy. Consider a patient with an overwhelmingly obvious injury – perhaps a broken wrist resembling the shape of a spoon. Would you consider the diagnostic process has been completed at that stage? You may be convinced of the diagnosis intuitively: the patient is in pain and saying his wrist is a funny shape and it certainly appears to lack anatomical normality. But what if this isn't the most important problem? What if the wrist injury is the result of fall caused by a brief giddy spell brought on by a sinister cardiac arrhythmia? Suddenly, this easy isolated diagnosis, made intuitively based on what you have seen, becomes a different issue. Seeing the injury has not provided understanding of the wider situation. You take the patient to the local minor injury unit where, on repeating the history of events to the triage nurse, the patient has another giddy turn and goes into cardiac arrest, with no access to a crash team. Leaping to the obvious conclusion that the broken wrist is the only thing wrong is one example of the many biases and fallacies humans succumb to when making decisions. Such assumptions and misconceptions, confidently presented to us in an assiduously truthful way by our subconscious, in fact steer us in the wrong direction. In this case, the presence of an obvious injury provided a **confirmation bias**. The writer Aldous Huxley (1894–1963) said 'facts do not cease to exist because they are ignored' (1927). While we don't intend to ignore things, many details are hidden (often in plain sight) and we must overcome the urge to leap intuitively to the easiest answer. This example of confirmation bias shows how we like to latch on to something tangible and convenient. The wrist fracture is easy to spot and diagnose clinically. The example highlights a purely intuitive approach, and one which shows how focusing on the '*what*' can lead to missing the '*why*'. It distracts from the need to continue to enquire and examine, to spot and to diagnose clinically. The potential for confirmation bias highlights the importance of good history taking, and we must be cautious about spending time screening patients using ECGs and other tests when they are not necessary.

So we now know that intuition on its own can be potentially problematic if it is not understood. Link it with experience and you can be in real trouble!

Experience

'I have been doing this job for 30 years, mate!'

There is a phenomenon that afflicts humans called the Dunning-Kruger Effect (Dunning and Kruger, 1999). It suggests that novices overstate their abilities, whereas experts understate their abilities and are at increased risk due to the extent of their exposure to that risk. Both groups are at risk because of their high levels of confidence, and Figure 5.1 demonstrates this. Based on the graph, one may believe that experience is favourable, and we are going to discuss this point to ensure that experience is approached cautiously using a very non-healthcare example.

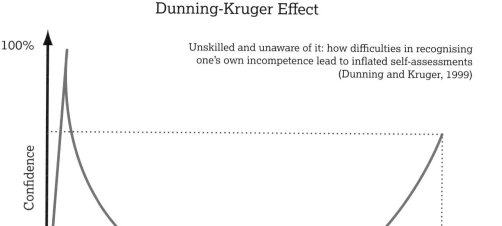

Figure 5.1: *The Dunning-Kruger Effect*

In extreme sports, such as BASE jumping[1], the statistics suggest the most (and presumably messiest) fatalities occur in those either new to the sport or those most experienced. The rookie stands at the top of a tall building and thinks 'How hard can this be?' He casts himself into space only to be blown back into the building causing a delay in his parachute opening and an inevitable sudden stop on the pavement below. The very experienced BASE jumper says 'I have done this jump 100 times – it must be OK' and also casts himself into space only to be hit by the novice as he plummets to earth landing next to him on the pavement. There is a middle order of people who are sufficiently experienced but who also have a magic ingredient – insight into their true ability – upon which they make sound decisions and judgements. This BASE jumper walks to the edge and thinks 'not this time – too windy' and goes for a drink, joining the rest of his friends in the bar who are mourning the loss of an old and dear friend, and that new guy!

This suggests therefore that there are stages of development that must be navigated and understood before experience is worth anything, and that newly acquired skills should be approached with modest self-deprecation rather than with exuberant hubris. There are seminal texts in healthcare literature which support this, and the book by Patricia Benner (*From Novice to Expert*) advocates the Dreyfus model (1980) which describes five stages in the progression from 'novice' to 'expert' in nursing practice:

1   BASE stands for Building, Antenna or Aerial, Span (bridge) and Earth, and involves jumping from them with a parachute.

- Novice;

- Advanced beginner;

- Competent;

- Proficient;

- Expert.

(Benner, 1984)

How do find your place on this scale? You may be reading this book as an undergraduate paramedic student, or a postgraduate moving into specialist or advanced practice. Regardless of where you think you are on the scale above, your place between novice and expert is only ever commensurate with your consolidated experience and competency, and your ability to apply introspection. This means that your career may feel like a game of snakes and ladders when you reassess yourself or as you move into a new level of practice. Developing this insight should actually improve your perception of yourself as a clinician and enhance your career by inspiring new career goals, and giving you aspirations to further improve the care you offer.

Building on this, there are other notable models which use steps in a scale, and which provide opportunities to assess yourself against the Dreyfus model. The steps in Table 5.1 can be aligned to the Dreyfus model, and support the basic principle that you need to assess your competence and abilities to ensure that you use your experience alongside your knowledge and insight in order to provide more certainty that you will come up with the correct answer.

Linked closely to the Dreyfus model are the four stages of competence associated with Abraham Maslow, although specific citation cannot be found in his major works. These four stages, referred to as Maslow's Hierarchy of Competence, describe very effectively the journey from novice to expert and also provides a place to reflect on the pitfalls of gaps in knowledge linked to overconfident, entirely experiential and intuitive decision making without the safety net of effective deductive reasoning, and provides a place to also ensure that any **illusory superiority** is challenged.

The Four Stages of Competence

Unconscious incompetence. The subject has no insight into their lack of understanding or skill. They may not place any value in the skill (for example, I don't believe in 12-lead ECG; 3-lead is fine) or be unwilling to learn, despite encouragement.

Conscious incompetence. The subject has the insight sufficient to recognise they do not have understanding or skill. They may want to learn new skills and have a will to resolve the knowledge gap.

Conscious competence. The subject knows they are capable of the skill, and understands it. They may not find it easy, and have to concentrate intently to achieve the outcome from the skill. The execution may lack fluency and flow, and appear deliberate.

Unconscious competence. The subject carries out the skill to such a degree as to be 'second nature'. Some psychomotor examples may be seen as 'muscle memory', and the subject may be able to do other tasks simultaneously. The subject is competent to the level of being able to teach others.

Score	Socrates/Rumsfeld*	Maslow
1	I don't know what I don't know	Unconsciously incompetent
2	I know what I don't know	Consciously incompetent
3	I know what I know	Consciously competent
4	I don't know what I know	Unconsciously competent

Table 5.1: *Levels of Expertise*

*This citation adapts and combines quotes by Socrates and Donald Rumsfeld (US Secretary of Defence, 1975-77 and 2001-06). Socrates defined the intellectually derived and respected 'Socratic Paradox', and Rumsfeld made a famously rambling speech which attempted to make a similar point.

By way of example, let's take three different paramedics and assess them for their place on the Novice to Expert scale, based on the steps in Table 5.1:

- Stacey is a newly qualified paramedic. She came top of her class and is now a registered healthcare professional. She passed the course, she gets to drive on blue lights and put cannulae into patients; she thinks she is invincible and that she has all the accumulated knowledge and skills needed for pre-hospital care.

- Jameel is a paramedic who qualified 15 years ago. He has 'been there, done that' and is the quintessentially unflappable clinician. He has seen hundreds of trauma cases, strokes and cardiac arrests. He knows when someone needs to go to hospital and when they don't.

- Will is halfway through his specialist paramedic course. He is learning (quickly) that the last 10 years have been spent dodging invisible bullets, and every new condition he learns about scares him.

Reflective Question

Where do you fit on the scale from Table 5.1: Levels of Expertise? Where would you plot yourself on the Dreyfus Scale? Can you relate this to any experiences you've had or decisions you've made in practice or on placement?

Think carefully about each feature and before reading on, make your own judgement on the cases of Stacey, Jameel and Will using the table below. Then add your own experiences in the row at the bottom.

Paramedic	Score from Table 5.1	Dreyfus Scale
Stacey		
Jameel		
Will		
You		

Table 5.2: Table for assessing examples on the Dreyfus Scale

How did you get on? Is there actually a correct answer to this? Perhaps not – so just compare your feelings to the answers in the completed table and consider the justifications given for each paramedic and see if you agree.

Paramedic	Score from Table 5.1	Dreyfus Scale	Justification
Stacey	1 – I don't know what I don't know	Novice	This paramedic is overconfident and thinks that there is no more to learn. She also lacks experience and consolidation in practice.
Jameel	1 – I don't know what I don't know	Advanced beginner	This paramedic has misplaced his experience for knowledge and has probably been lucky so far, rather than skilful.

Paramedic	Score from Table 5.1	Dreyfus Scale	Justification
Will	2 - I know what I don't know	Novice	This paramedic has reset the clocks and gone back to school to become a specialist paramedic. In this context he is a novice again, but he has the insight to know what he doesn't know.
Your self-assessment			

Table 5.3: *Assessment of the scenarios using the Dreyfus Scale*

This exercise is an oversimplification, but highlights the fact that the experience does not necessarily confer competency.

When it comes to experience, you will meet colleagues on your travels who make statements extolling their brilliance by dint of decades of experience – 'I have been doing this job for 30 years, mate' or similar assertions, usually peppered with embellished tales of 'derring-do'. Without wanting to denigrate 30 years of dedicated service to patients, it is still appropriate to ask what those 30 years meant in reality. Let's put it this way: if you walk to work using the same route every day for a year, can you say you have an extra year's worth of experience of making journeys on foot? Could you therefore infer from this experience that this made you a better walker or navigator? Of course not. You have simply walked the same walk dozens of times following on from the very first day when you learned the route. Similarly, make sure that you can account for your clinical experiences by satisfying yourself that you haven't repeated the same one over and over without learning from it. Experience requires consolidation and learning before you even consider applying it intuitively. Even then, relying on intuition is risky.

In the film *Groundhog Day,* the character Phil (played by Bill Murray) has been given a gift from which all clinicians would benefit once in their careers. He is able to completely mess up every experience on that given day, time and time and time again, each time trying something different to improve the outcome. For instance, he had no idea that Rita likes French poetry – how could he have known on day one? After several attempts though he learns a poem which captivates her, thereby moving her emotionally towards his ultimate goal. This play on how experience is gained and consolidated is a great example for clinicians – particularly when you contrast the intuitive approach Phil takes early on in the film with his later actions. As he gains experience, he learns what works and what doesn't.

Experience, therefore, is useful rather than essential. We should try to quantify what experience is when we consider relying on it. Remember the pitfalls that come with using intuition or experience in isolation. When standing on the precipice of a clinical decision that will affect a real-life patient, that is more complex than you realise. Imagine yourself as the BASE jumper. Are you going to jump today because it was OK on the previous one hundred emergency calls, or do you use your experience to think of other options?

Hypotheses: Developing and Testing Ideas

This final section provides an overview of the function of hypotheses, and how to make deductions based upon them. In clinical care, hypotheses can include a list of differential diagnoses – the list of conditions which are possible in the presence of the signs and symptoms the patient has, and upon which each must be considered and tested in order to exclude them. In much the same way when playing Cluedo, if you have the Professor Plum card in your hand, he cannot be the murderer and you can absolutely exclude him.

As we suggested in the previous section, experience isn't absolutely essential, and a lack of it does not need to hamper your practice. People who lack experience can develop good hypotheses if they use a good decision-making method. The literature shows that novices are just as able to develop hypotheses, but it does take them longer to identify them. By way of an example, imagine your car won't start and you don't have breakdown cover. You are not a qualified mechanic, you are a total novice. There are a number of things that even a lay person can resolve to bring a car back to life, so before you even lift the bonnet you begin to make a list of things you are aware of and plan to work your way through them:

- Is there enough fuel?
- Is the battery flat?
- If the car has one, did you turn the immobiliser (anti-theft device) off?

You start with the battery. The engine turns over quickly but won't fire, so the battery isn't flat. That hypothesis has been excluded absolutely. Now to the fuel – is there enough? The fuel gauge is showing as full, so there is enough fuel. Another hypothesis springs to mind – is it the correct fuel? You check your petrol station receipt and what you put in last night matches your vehicle's fuel type – we can exclude that. Check the immobiliser next. Push the button on the key fob and the light doesn't flash. This is looking likely, so you go back in the house and get your partner's key ring and return to the car. Push the button on the key fob and try the key – the car starts. This simple example works in clinical care scenarios too and highlights the importance of making enquiry, developing, testing and excluding hypotheses within the scope of your knowledge. What if the car had a major problem with its ignition system which the owner couldn't possibly fix? They would have phoned a garage for advice with a view to getting a mechanic to take a look at it. If the clinician cannot find out what is wrong with a patient, they too can get advice and refer the patient. Sometimes it is OK to not know, and admitting you don't know is always preferable to guessing and hoping for the best. This will affect the outcome of the Garden Path Test!

Let's look at a somewhat simplified clinical scenario which highlights how you can exclude conditions by testing the hypotheses. (The scenario in the box assumes a more complete history taking and physical examination has taken place, and has been shortened to highlight the testing of each main hypothesis.)

Case Scenario: Laura

You are called to a 17-year-old female with abdominal pain. She is in her room accompanied by her mother. She complains of diffuse abdominal discomfort and nausea. She is usually fit and well and has an active social life.

You immediately start to draw on your knowledge (and experience, in this case) to consider some of the possible common conditions.

- Appendicitis;
- Gastroenteritis;
- Pregnancy;
- Renal colic;
- Pelvic inflammatory disease.

You ask questions relevant to each of these:

'Do you have your appendix?' The patient had her appendix out as a child – so not appendicitis.

'Any diarrhoea or vomiting, and has anyone else been ill in the family?' She has no diarrhoea or vomiting, just slight nausea for two days. So it's not gastroenteritis either.

'Could you be pregnant?' Laura's mother says unequivocally that she could not be, and why have you asked. (Interesting …)

'Could I test your urine please?' The patient asks if that includes a pregnancy test. (More interesting …)

The urine test shows that Laura is pregnant. You are worried that her pain is a complication of early pregnancy and explain gently that you need to send her to hospital.

(Laura's case is also used in more detail in the next chapter.)

Abdominal pain is a good example to use as it is notoriously difficult to get the diagnosis correct. In fact the literature suggests that you should expect to be wrong with your diagnosis 50% of the time (Simon et al., 2005). The most important point is that the process of making the correct decision must be used and you cannot simply walk away based on a hunch (intuition) or based on pattern recognition only (experience). If the patient in the example above had been assessed using only intuition or experience, she might have been left at home with a potentially life-threatening condition.

Charlin et al. (2000) suggest that decision making based on information processing is made utilising cycles of hypotheses and deduction in an iterative way, building and testing hypotheses from many sources. The case study involving Laura demonstrates the cyclical nature of decision making and the importance of using process. It is important to know where to get the information from, and recognise the sources you can use to generate hypotheses. Arguably, there is no such thing as an inappropriate hypothesis, but as you become more practised in decision-making process you will pre-select hypotheses worthy of testing. For example, in most textbooks the list of differential diagnoses for abdominal pain includes pregnancy/ectopic pregnancy as a cause, but of course if your patient is male you can discount this as a hypothesis. You may also choose to exclude this hypothesis in female children under a certain age, women who have undergone hysterectomy, or women clearly beyond childbearing age.

So, what sources of information can be used to generate your hypotheses? The main groups can be broken down into different lines of enquiry, such as:

- What the patient tells you;
- What the patient chooses not to tell you;
- What family members and carers tell you;
- Signs (i.e. skin colour);
- Symptoms (i.e. nausea);
- Diagnostic tests (i.e. ECG, blood glucose, blood pressure).

For example, a patient tells you he has had some episodes of chest pain. He doesn't tell you that actually it's been going on for some days, and his wife says she is worried. The patient is pale and clammy and complains of feeling sick. His ECG does not show any acute changes, but his blood pressure is raised. Clearly the hypotheses will include myocardial infarction and acute coronary syndrome, but they may also include hernia, peptic ulcer, and stress. Each of these hypotheses need to be tested to ensure that the patient has the correct care pathway. It is almost inevitable that you won't be able to find the formal diagnosis at the patient's side because blood tests will be necessary to assess cardiac enzymes. You have tested your hypotheses and reached the point where you can enquire no more.

In any scenario, this process can be repeated until you reach a point where you either find the answer, or you decide that you are unable to find the answer – your capability point. The graph in Figure 5.2 shows how you start with many hypotheses and, as you move towards the solution, the number of hypotheses reduces. Eventually, either one correct answer will remain, or you will have reached the red line at which point you must refer to someone else.

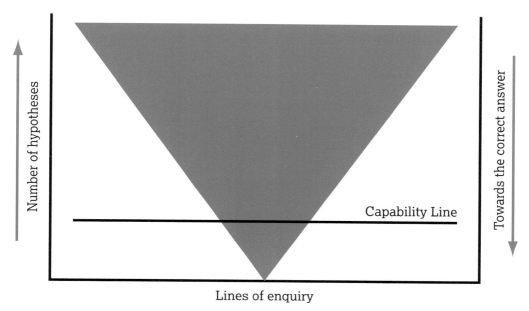

Figure 5.2: Hypotheses and solutions line

Conclusion

Passing the Garden Path Test requires you to have made a robust decision which can be defended and explained. While the origins of the test arose from a scenario involving leaving a patient at home and not sending them to hospital, every decision has a garden path regardless of the complexity of the scenario or acuity of the patient. The outcome of the test hinges on making sure you have addressed the 'why' as well as 'what', and that any decisions stand up to your own reflective scrutiny.

There will always be times where you simply do not know what is wrong with the patient. Until such time as there are portable CT scanners and integrated point of care blood tests available, you will have to refer the patient for ongoing care to another clinical team. Bear in mind that the decision to refer patients is a decision in itself, and must be approached with the same consideration.

Remember that you can use peers and senior colleagues to test your hypotheses, and the process of shared decision making is a very good way of enhancing patient safety. Do not mistake your autonomy as a pressure to work alone. Autonomy gives you freedom to think and freedom to act, and choosing to seek advice and guidance does not make you a bad clinician and should not make you feel less autonomous. However, abdicating your decision making and sending all your patients to hospital would suggest a lack of autonomy and professional responsibility.

As you move from this chapter into the next, consider the decisions you make and the conclusions you draw. Think about the importance of each decision point – the fork in the road requiring taking a particular route – and how difficult it is to track back once you have negotiated three or four major decisions in a row. The fact is that making good decisions is good for patients, and developing your professional practice means taking responsibility. Decision-making skills require practice. You will move from novice to expert as long as you know what you know, and what you don't know.

Professional Practice and Learning Pointers

This chapter set out to guide you through the basic principles of decision making, based on gaining a better understanding of the components involved. The use of intuition and experience in isolation was discussed, and the introduction of ways to understand what you know and what you don't know has been presented. The use of hypotheses and how you test them in order to deduce answers has been reviewed as the final piece of the puzzle. The next chapter looks in more detail at the theories that underpin these concepts, and introduces the **cognitive continuum** and a more in-depth assessment of how to obtain data and assess its accuracy. This is an important aspect in practice as it means that you will approach practice in a safe and professional way.

Reflective Exercises

- Pick a clinical condition you think you know well and try to develop a list of signs and symptoms which are associated with the condition. Then develop a list of hypotheses to test.

- Reflect on the use of intuition in your personal and professional life. Consider when it matters and when it doesn't. Then consider times where you have acted intuitively – regardless of the outcome being correct or incorrect – and review your processing.

- How do you perceive experience in practice? Reflecting on the novice to expert journey, how important is experience in comparison to effective structured decision making?

6 The Cognitive Continuum: Enhancing your Decision Making Skills

Chapter Objectives

This chapter will cover:

- Defining the cognitive continuum;
- Information processing;
- Professional judgements;
- Converting experience into hypothesis development;
- Mitigating risk: management versus avoidance.

Introduction

This chapter looks in more detail at drawing together the individual decision-making processes and concepts and links them into a single system which can both improve the way you make decisions, and make care safer for your patients. Please read the clinical scenario before embarking on the chapter as it will be used throughout the chapter as a point of reference to help illustrate some of the areas discussed.

Case Scenario: Laura

You are called to a 17-year-old female complaining of abdominal pain. The patient lives with her parents in a very affluent part of town and is accompanied by her boyfriend and her mother.

You establish the chief complaint and reason for calling 999 as worsening lower abdominal pain. The history leading to the 999 call is two days of abdominal discomfort. You manage to elicit that she is not expecting to menstruate for another two weeks and that she is not experiencing bleeding Per Vagina.

The patient is asked if she is sexually active, and her mother states categorically that she is not before she has a chance to answer. Her boyfriend chooses not to comment. She has no reported medication history, but you specifically ask about oral contraception as some patients do not consider this as medicine. She denies taking the oral contraceptive pill. Her observations are as follows:

Heart Rate	118 regular
Respiratory rate	14 (inspiration noted as being limited by discomfort)
Blood pressure	105/68
Temperature	37.0°
BM	5.4 mmol

Table 6.1: Laura's observations

Her abdomen is unremarkable on inspection, auscultation and percussion but tender to light palpation in the lower quadrants. She had no rebound tenderness and is negative to **Rovsing's test; obturator sign** and **psoas sign.** She is also negative to **Murphy's sign.**

You are uncomfortable with the evidence given in the history and you are concerned about simply discharging the patient with a diagnosis of non-specific abdominal pain. You seek consent to screen the patient's urine for abnormality and specifically state that this will include a pregnancy test. The patient becomes very anxious about the pregnancy test but consents. The urinalysis shows blood +++ and the **bHCG test** is positive.

With this evidence, you are confident in a diagnosis of pregnancy with potential early signs of the pregnancy being ectopic. You duly admit the patient to the local hospital.

Defining the Cognitive Continuum

The cognitive continuum theory was created by Kenneth Hammond from the University of Colorado in 1981, and has its origins in psychology rather than healthcare. The initial theory was transposed into a health perspective in the late 1980s by Robert Hamm from the University of Oklahoma. Hamm (1988) pulled together the component theories of deduction and intuition into a single process with six modes of enquiry ranging from pure science at one extreme to pure intuition at the other (Figure 6.1). Decision making moving around the middle ground in this gradient is known as **quasi-rationality** ('quasi' = resembling and 'rationality' = with reason). Quasi-rationality is the product of the application of the cognitive continuum – eliciting the decision based on a blend of intuition and cognition – and requires the user to process accurate and appropriate hypotheses. The six modes of enquiry described by Hamm have clear demarcation, and yet the decision making needs to move on a sliding scale up and down the cognitive continuum. This is particularly true in the paramedic practice setting, where clinicians have access to science (such as blood tests) and absolute intuition (**heuristics**). Decisions can be made at the poles of cognitive continuum theory and may therefore lack either intuition or analysis. But for the most part the bounded reality of quasi-rationality provides the basis for decisions to be made based on prevailing availability of factors, or the seeking of further evidence to refer to and test.

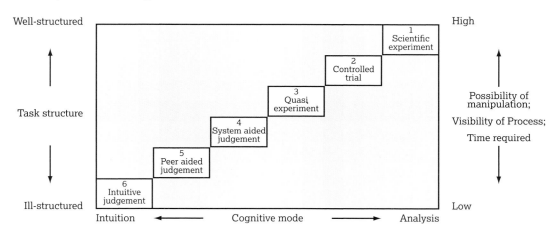

Figure 6.1: *Six Modes of Enquiry (Hamm, 1988)*

Many of the studies undertaken into decision-making methods suggest that clinicians in their early years of practice choose either intuition or analysis, often based on their educational background or the influence of senior colleagues and supervisors. As practice develops and experience emerges, more trust is often placed in intuition. Limited empirical support is sought, and often only achieved tacitly. As professional practice develops, we should look forward using reasoning, but we may retain a more novice approach which does not keep pace with time in practice, and which tends to look back on experiences to achieve a decision. Experience is often regarded as a strong currency in healthcare roles. While more experienced clinicians can generate hypotheses more rapidly and easily, the deductive ability is no more effective in the expert practitioner than the novice. The expert user of the cognitive continuum is able to move fluidly within it; gaining new information, testing, retesting, validating and rejecting information dynamically – demonstrating further that experience and skill in processing information can contribute to more effective decision making. When used dynamically, the cognitive continuum is like the game Snakes and Ladders – making progress towards a decision only to lose ground rapidly on the next roll of the dice.

Clinical judgement based on sound decision making as an overarching concept can be described as the ability to apply a quasi-rational decision to the balance of analysis/cognition and intuition. Arguably, to use the cognitive continuum effectively, the clinician must have a certain level of ability in their knowledge domain, a minimum level of competency in practice, and a level of experience sufficient to confidently approach the problem. However, experience only speeds up the generation of hypotheses and their specificity.

Information Processing

Diagnosis is one of the cornerstones of the technical aspect of clinical practice. It provides patients with information about their symptoms, disease trajectory and recovery. Reaching a diagnosis in practice is little more than an exercise in categorisation – recognising or comparing something against a known control. The way we make decisions is covered extensively throughout this book, and we have discussed the two main ways we as humans make decisions (System 1 – fast/ intuitive; System 2 – slow/deliberate) (Kahneman, 2011). This section looks at decision making based on information processing, utilising cycles of hypothesis and deduction in an iterative way, building and testing hypotheses. Information is usually gained from a range of sources (for instance, the patient's long-term history, their onset of illness, and other information such as physiological markers like blood pressure). The concept of the Information Processing Model, which examines the way decision makers rationally identify and test theories and hypotheses, is very much associated with the model employed by medicine. It has begun to emerge as the systematic methodology used by paramedics to ensure that the correct decisions are made. It also contributes to developing treatment plans and referral or discharge decisions. Being able to find information and process it effectively provides the clues within the dilemmas we face in practice. These in turn become hypotheses needed to help solve the problem. This is a vitally important aspect of the decision-making skill of clinicians.

There is a basic four stage deductive process which was first described by Radwin in 1990, and Hamers et al. in 1994 was a more accessible and simplified version of the more detailed seven stage process described by Carnevali et al. in 1984. Both models effectively demonstrate the steps that decision makers must take to accurately reach the correct answer. Of course, these theories assume that the information being considered is correct in the first place. The father of the computer, Charles Babbage (b 1791, d 1871), was once asked:

> *'Pray, Mr. Babbage, if you put into the machine wrong figures, will the right answers come out?'*
>
> *(Babbage, 1864)*

His response to the question was far from polite by all accounts. He hadn't considered that anyone would put in the wrong information, or perhaps that his machine was not capable of correcting these errors. Either way, the fact remains that if you put the wrong information in, the wrong answer is almost inevitable. In the last chapter, we looked at human factors and how the subject emerged from the experiences and adverse incidents from the aviation industry. Think about the WHO surgical checklist and how this prevented significant errors by 50% almost overnight. Much of the essence of the checklist is the need to sense check (process) the information before using it. For example, asking the patient which leg they are expecting to wake up with has prevented mistaken amputations. By way of contrast, in the aviation industry a notable negative event where information was incorrectly processed was the Kegworth Air Crash in January 1989. The aircraft suffered an engine fire in one engine, and because the pilot could smell smoke through the air conditioning he assumed he could shut down the engine which runs the air conditioning. If he had checked he would have realised that, on the 400 series Boeing 737, the air conditioning is run from the opposite engine than the one it is run from in the 300 series with which he was very familiar. He shut down the good engine by mistake, and then failed to understand why this action didn't resolve the problem – ultimately leading to the crash and the loss of 47 lives. The loss of one engine on a modern airliner is an inconvenience rather than a disaster, but poor information processing and making assumptions led to a disaster.

In the computing industry, poor information processing has evolved into the modern acronym of 'GIGO' – garbage in, garbage out. This has lots of applications in health decision making (and aviation). If we accept the earlier statement that deduction is no more than categorisation or computation, the risk of inputting the wrong information and expecting the correct answer to come out must arguably be the greatest pitfall of the decision maker. It also has strong links with the decision to trust your old brain or your new brain (system 1/system 2) and allowing intuition to drive you (which engine will you shut down if you don't think about it?) Looking back to where we considered the use of intuition as a useful tool in creating ideas, we should be mindful that creating hypotheses is a psychological necessity. There is nothing worse than staring at something with no idea what to do. This doesn't occur where you achieve an initial intuitive feeling as this provides reassurance and a base upon which to build the decision-making case – but it isn't the way to find the final answer. Information processing, like all aspects of decision making, is an active process and the processing is simply an assessment of probability, based on evidence or experience. (For example, if you have Professor Plum in your hand of cards when playing Cluedo, he isn't the murderer.) The information you select as ideas or hypotheses must themselves be validated to avoid correct processing of incorrect data.

The default approach, particularly in diagnostic reasoning, involves deductive reasoning rather than reliance on pure intuition. As previously discussed, however, this must not be at the expense of decisiveness in an emergency. It is important to recognise the utility of intuition when discussing hypothetico-deduction, as the information upon which deduction is based is usually derived from intuitive, experiential, or (in the worst-case scenario) tacit knowledge. Healthcare decision making often requires significant evidence of knowledge and competency – particularly in relation to the knowledge of health, disease and therapy. Clinicians, therefore, need confidence as well as competence in order to operate effectively and safely. The development of the decision-making skills is no different to learning about the diseases or treatments faced in practice.

In the scenario described at the start of the chapter, the data acquisition and processing phase elicits many statements upon which the initial hypothesis was formed. There are however compounding factors which would have had a negative impact had this been overlooked. Decision makers should remain open minded and be prepared to step back when processing information in dynamic and high-pressure environments, or where experience in a particular area of practice is still in development. (This is different to the perception of those not chronologically experienced.) The evidence shows that where clinicians lack experience, their practice is no less safe but decisions may not be made as rapidly. This is due to the time needed to process data, create and test hypotheses.

Before moving on, let's think back to the previous chapter where the concepts of human factors and bias were discussed.

In the scenario involving Laura (described at the start of the chapter), the denial of sexual activity may have closed the line of questioning and examination leading to the actual diagnosis. It would have given rise to a false conclusion, supporting the deductive process of decision making. This illustrates the point that decisions should be based on sound, validated information – *garbage in, garbage out.* We assume that the patient tells the truth, even when they do not (perhaps their own truth), and therefore **positivism** in the context of aspects such as moral judgements in history taking may lead to false information being given (denial of sexual activity leading to exclusion of obstetric causes of abdominal pain). Health professionals should perhaps avoid being cynical in front of patients, but should be open minded and take a **post-positivist** approach, particularly when taking a patient's history.

Often the initial hypothesis may be the strongest or most obvious and become the final diagnosis. It is therefore important to remember not to fall back on judgement based on its outcome and its use of intuition, as this puts us back to be driven by 'what', rather than 'why'. In the case given, the strong, most obvious hypothesis was generated intuitively based on the clinical presentation, age and gender of the patient. That embedded heuristic information had to be processed to avoid placing unwarranted faith in what appeared obvious (do we always know what we don't know?) Consider what may have happened if the patient's mother's denial, and the patient's own lack of opposition to this, had been accepted at face value. Potentially, this lack of information processing and selection of a reasonable hypothesis to test could have been life threatening. Decision making is a dynamic process which is based on making choices and judgements. Deliberation – careful consideration of each step taken prior to arriving at a decision or a diagnosis – is important if the patient's best interests are to be secured.

Professional Judgements

It is sadly more common to reflect on examples where judgement was poor, usually arising from an error or omission in practice, sometimes involving a patient suffering harm. Professional practice implies that a range of considerations are required to uphold patient safety, experience and outcomes. Judgements are formed considering the knowledge and skills possessed, and their application judiciously considered. The most common assessment of professional judgement arises in the context of the responsibility with which professionals are entrusted in their day-to-day work. Professional judgements are at the heart of practice and are at the sharp end of each phase of care, intervention, plan, dilemma, conversation, and approach to risk.

One of the more common pieces of advice given to paramedics in training – particularly in previous decades – is the notion of 'if in doubt, don't' (or, indeed, 'if in doubt, do'). The belief that defaults and axioms are acceptable judgements is outmoded and has no place in modern healthcare, let alone paramedic practice. Consider a scenario relating to the application of CPR in a patient with a Do Not Attempt Cardiopulmonary Resuscitation (DNACPR) instruction, where the document cannot be located. Every family member agrees it exists, the GP on the end of the telephone confirms that he signed it, and there is an advance directive signed by the patient in their community care record. Following the advice 'if in doubt, do', the presence of doubt may drive the clinician to apply CPR regardless of knowing that this is not what the patient wanted, and that it will be futile – the act being perceived perhaps in terms of self-preservation based on a false perception of punitive action being likely. The advice perhaps should always be 'if in doubt, make a decision'. Decisions and professional judgements that are well made, defensible and not associated with professional jeopardy, should be relied upon. In the DNACPR scenario given, the judgement to not resuscitate is based on the balance of information and the cognitive approach to the final decision. The patient is suffering the end stage of their disease, their treatment regime is palliative, the family are aware that their relative's demise is imminent, and so on. The professional judgement is yours to make, and the outcome should not cloud the focus on the importance of doing the correct thing. The nature of making professional judgements and the importance of understanding why they need to be made is a particular aspect of decision-making psychology which must be logical and cognitive, rather than rash and emotional.

A theme which runs through clinical practice is the need to practise defensibly, rather than defensively. Defensive practice is associated with clinician-centred, rather than patient-centred care and fails to consider the crucial nature of the role of the caregiver in healthcare. It is useful to consider your professional judgements in the context of the NHS '6Cs':

- Care;
- Compassion;
- Courage;
- Communication;
- Commitment;
- Competence.

(NHS England, 2014a)

Converting Experience into Hypothesis Development

As previously discussed, experience (chronological or episodic) is not absolutely essential in the formation of hypotheses, but experience in practice does serve to speed up the process of hypothesis generation. Remembering that creating a hypothesis is not in itself a decision, hypothesis generation is arguably a good place to allow your intuition to be exploited. Hypotheses are usually 'whats' without the 'whys' and will be tested as part of the deductive process. Therefore a hypothesis is a good place to make assumptions, safe in the knowledge that no idea is taken forward without it first being 'sense checked' (information processing) and/or deductively accepted or rejected. For example, the patient with the shortened and rotated leg following a fall in a care home is most likely to have a broken hip, except if they have already had a total hip replacement, in which case the injury is more likely to be related to damage to the prosthesis. If you fail to test the hypothesis (history, examination of area of injury) the chances of being right goes right back to intuition, and while on occasions the answer may be correct, the outcome of the decision is poor because it was only correct in hindsight.

Generating the list of hypotheses may be in the form of a list of differential diagnoses, and therefore may be taken from existing literature or guidance. It may need relatively little knowledge of the diseases listed, or at least be far less structured. An example of this may be in patients displaying challenging behaviour. Intuitively, the assumption may be that this is an acute mental health emergency linked to primary psychiatric pathology, but when you look at the possible list of reasons someone may have altered behaviour the list extends significantly beyond mental health. For example, it might include:

- Psychoactive drugs
- Sepsis
- Alzheimer's disease
- Meningitis
- **Encephalitis**
- HIV-associated **encephalopathy**
- Brain tumours
- Head injuries
- Multiple sclerosis
- Parkinson disease
- Seizure disorders
- Stroke
- Kidney failure
- Liver failure

- Hypoglycaemia
- Lupus
- Hypothyroidism
- Hyperthyroidism.

When categorising these, the context of the behaviour becomes important. For example, does the patient also have:

- Confusion or delirium
- Delusions
- Disorganised speech or behaviour
- Hallucinations
- Mood extremes (such as depression)?

A consistent theme throughout this book is the importance of approaching decisions based on structured enquiry, using methods to test, retest, reject or accept each theory considering dynamically how other complex factors drive the process that leads to the correct outcome. Consider then how dismissing a patient with challenging behaviour on the basis of *what* they are outwardly displaying could lead to a poor outcome and experience for the patient. Again, considering that diagnosis is a categorisation task, miscategorising patients' needs becomes ethically questionable. So the hypothesis becomes ever more important as a step on the way to the decision you make, and therefore subsequent onward decisions for treatment, referral etc.

As with all things that involve human beings, we can be wrong – even if we use the correct approach, process and methods.

Mitigating Risk: Management vs Avoidance

Healthcare is a risky business. Patients deserve the very best care and this must be delivered in a safe way. It is simply unrealistic though to manage every condition by referring to a hospital consultant or putting the patient through a barrage of tests. Most health conditions that occur spontaneously (illness) or are acquired (injury) are self-limiting, or need only minor interventions to correct, but some are cryptic, occult, atypical, or overlaid upon a complex health history. For some patients, illness and injury are compounded by extremes of age, social and economic circumstance, or capacity to care for oneself. Against this backdrop, we are expected to reduce the impact on our wider health and social care systems.

> ## Manage risk
>
> ### Identify and minimise risks
>
> You must take all reasonable steps to reduce the risk of harm to service users, carers and colleagues as far as possible.
>
> You must not do anything, or allow someone else to do anything, which could put the health or safety of a service user, carer or colleague at unacceptable risk.

Figure 6.2: *Managing risk (from HCPC, 2016)*

Safe care is not about taking risks, it is about understanding risks and seeking to mitigate as far as is reasonable. Sadly, things do not always run to plan and patients can deteriorate unexpectedly or suffer a new, separate health emergency. When this happens – particularly when it leads on to an investigation – it can have a deleterious effect on the confidence of the clinician who last cared for the patient whose outcome wasn't favourable, as well as the patient.

Looking back to the biomedical ethics section in Chapter 2, there is an adaptation of the Kantian quote which states that the patient must only ever be the end, and never a means to an end. This applies when taking baggage away from a previous encounter, and while it is important to reflect and learn from previous encounters and errors, care must be taken to avoid taking the circumstances on to the next patient contact; ensuring that events do not have a negative effect on team or organisational culture. Examples exist from ambulance services where entire groups of staff change their practice in the wake of a colleague being investigated, increasing the number of patients taken to hospital on the basis of the anxiety generated by what is entirely separate and removed from their own practice. This social phenomenon is not unique to ambulance services, and exists across all paramedic practice settings, healthcare in general, and probably in other industries in their own context too.

Chapter 5 is called 'The Garden Path Test', and discusses the ways in which we can avoid accumulating unresolved concerns resulting from bad decisions. Making a good decision must also include mitigation against error, and there are strategies which can be used to help underpin each encounter to ensure your patient is safe, and your practice is not influenced by fear – rather it is bounded by an understanding of risks, and is resolved in such a way that protects all concerned as far as possible.

Step 1 on this process is shared or collaborative decision making – making sure patients understand what you have found, what you are proposing to do, and what might happen next. Seeking understanding from your patient (where their capacity allows) greatly enhances the approach to risk. While decisions made with a patient must be done in light of good information (and that responsibility ultimately sits with the clinician), the patient who understands and consents to the course of action is the first line of defence regarding anticipated issues and ensuring they seek help.

It would be unwise to omit reference to the patients for whom capacity is diminished, and the occasions where decisions are made in the best interest of a patient. The hypothetico-deductive model may be affected by the patient's capacity to understand questions. On occasion this may lead to a more clinically diagnostic approach, rather than through considering the health history primarily. For example, the unconscious patient cannot tell you why they are unconscious, and may not have any clues about their person to guide the decision. Therefore, you look to the common causes as hypotheses (hypoglycaemia, intoxication etc.) and exclude or confirm accordingly. Where the cause is hypoglycaemia, a blood glucose test can be obtained (in the patient's best interest) to confirm the cause, and this then allows treatment to be focused. This is a very simple example of capacity being diminished acutely and temporarily, and it is important that clinicians understand the principles associated with decision making involving patients who may lack capacity. There are many resources that can be accessed relating to this topic, including:

- The Mental Capacity Act (2005)
- Making decisions: A guide for people who work in health and social care
- Mental Capacity Act 2005 – Code of Practice

One of the most important aspects of risk mitigation is documentation. Making a contemporaneous record of each healthcare encounter is essential in ensuring what happened was recorded and can be revisited in the future as necessary. It is a commonly used quotation that always bears repeating:

If it isn't written down, it didn't happen.

Keep records of your work

Keep accurate records

You must keep full, clear, and accurate records for everyone you care for, treat, or provide other service to.

You must complete all records promptly and as soon as possible after providing care, treatment or other services.

Figure 6.3: Keeping records of your work (taken from HCPC, 2016)

The prospect of managing risk can be somewhat daunting and it is important that clinicians develop clear strategies to ensure that the responsibility of professional practice doesn't overwhelm or create unnecessary pressure, which may in turn lead to worse care for the patient. There is a significant difference between defensible practice and defensive practice, and the methods you choose to use to promote safe practice for your patient and yourself should be proportional.

- *Defensive*
  - Used or intended to defend or protect.
  - Very anxious to challenge or avoid criticism.
- *Defensible*
  - Justifiable by argument.
  - Able to be protected.

Many of the synonyms associated with the word defensible are common to decision making, such as; *justifiable, arguable, tenable, defendable, maintainable, sustainable, supportable, plausible, well founded, sound, sensible, reasonable, rational, logical.*

Structured documentation will help you to defend your practice, should this ever be necessary. More importantly it ensures that you prevent harm coming to your patient. Therefore, perhaps instead of perceiving the aspects of practice you employ to 'cover yourself', change your perspective and view these activities as those which make your care as safe as possible for your patient. For paramedics, and in fact all healthcare professionals, discharging a patient from care is probably the activity which carries the greatest perception of risk by clinicians, and is the reason the 'Garden Path Test' was developed. It is a fact that some patients will worsen, and/or the diagnosis/treatment given was incorrect. To err is human, and while we have argued in this book that diagnosis is merely a categorisation task, sometimes even the best clinicians make errors. Therefore, it is not the act of discharging a patient in good faith and with adequate safety netting that represents the most risk – it is failing to consider the worst-case scenario and mitigating against it.

There are many models for structuring documentation, and some Trusts provide pre-formatted and/or pre-printed patient advice leaflets to support the advice given verbally to patients. The following headings are a suggested format for structuring written clinical records. These headings can be completed concisely, and need not take very long, but must cover the key areas discussed with the patient. Remember, these headings should reflect a conversation with the patient, and not exist solely as documentation in isolation.

Worsening Care Advice (WCA)

This is a list of 'what ifs' – the signs and symptoms which may be encountered by the patient (or witnessed by friends of family) and which may then require a follow up action, which should also be documented and communicated to the patient/family/carer.

For example, a patient who has back pain should expect the pain to remain quite constant and ease gradually over the coming days. The WCA discussed with the patient would involve a change to the pattern of pain, and include the red flags for Cauda Equina.

Safety Netting

Safety Netting was introduced into Primary Care some years ago, and lacks a consensus on what it must include. Therefore, the suggestion to use it in combination with WCA and Left in Care of (see below) is an interpretation of its application in practice which focuses on the specific 'what to do' advice in response to the Worsening Care Advice.

For example, the patient with back pain should be advised that if they still have pain in several weeks (as is common with non-traumatic back pain) they should approach their GP. However, if they experience the signs and symptoms of Cauda Equina, they should seek urgent follow up immediately. Safety Netting may be specific and include calling 111 or 999.

Left in Care of (LICO)

This aspect of this format of documentation records who will be caring for the patient in the immediate period after their discharge (or while waiting for referral). While for some patients this won't be necessary, and for some it won't be an option, where a friend, carer or neighbour is prepared to provide some after-care, it is important to document this, and include the patient's consent for this to happen.

For example, you may document 'Left in care of neighbour who will sit with the patient until their daughter arrives. The patient has consented to this, and the WCA has been discussed with them'.

Structured documentation is a contemporaneous record of the encounter with you and your patient, and while it may never again see the light of day after the day it was written, it remains a part of the patient's health record and is retained for at least 10 years for adults, and many more years for children. Remember to make your written records well structured, and use them to promote patient safety as a record of what you have advised your patient. This applies in all practice settings and, while it is most important when ending an episode of care (as opposed to taking a patient to the emergency department), consistent structured clinical documentation is a practised skill, which healthcare professionals must consider a cornerstone of practice that keeps patients safe and clinicians confident.

Conclusion

Good decision making promotes the best possible outcomes for patients (Muir, 2004). The use of intuition is an essential aspect of decision making. It is used by the expert decision maker to frame their experiences in the context of processing new information identified, leading to good hypotheses generation. This promotes the use of deduction, and allows for more rapid and accurate decisions to be made. The cognitive continuum provides a deductive cycle, which provides practitioners with the opportunity to challenge and re-challenge their thinking and promotes safe and reproducible decision making in practice. Moreover, the components of the cognitive continuum could be considered as operating antagonistically or cyclically; intuition can provide the early warning or prompt, which the hypothetico-deductive process needs to confound or support. Conversely, the interpretation of pure deduction of hypotheses can be challenged with intuition, based on experts' epistemological awareness of expected truths.

In emergency and urgent care, paramedics must now be able to identify positively that a patient is not seriously ill and to signpost effectively, rather than passing the patient onto the Emergency Department to make further decisions. In the scenario described, the information which was processed was challenged and re-processed leading to the correct outcome. Decision making is an active process at all ends of the acuity spectrum and links closely to the way risk is identified, stratified and mitigated. Paramedics must be prepared for the situations where they hear hooves and see zebras – and to accept that sometimes those zebras will quack!

The next and final chapter is a series of case studies intended to highlight exactly the pitfalls described in the contents of this book, and provides a practical breakdown of the elements we have discussed in other chapters to highlight where we make errors because of our basic human fallibilities. This isn't a psychology textbook. Rather, it aims to prompt and challenge you to think critically, be more sceptical of yourself, process information, hypothesise, deduce, and decide. Consider if you will the Cocktail Party Effect – the ability to single out a voice in a noisy room while having a conversation with someone. If you hear someone else say your name, your brain picks this out seamlessly from the cacophony of other voices. Without conscious thought, imagine what we miss every day, and in every encounter with our patients.

Reflective Exercises

- Consider the importance of risk management and mitigation and how you might approach this while ensuring the patient's interest remains paramount, and does not become 'the means to an end'.

- Using the principles of the Cognitive Continuum, think of a time when you knew the answer to a simple diagnosis (i.e. clinical diagnosis of a fractured neck of femur from its classic signs – shortening and external rotation of the affected leg).

Reflect on how you came to the decision and consider any compounding factors which may affect the diagnosis (there are only a few!).

- Thinking back to the Humpty Dumpty exercise in Chapter 3, consider a situation where the information you used was taken at face value. Undertake a reflective cycle which used the principles of Information Processing to change the decision, or improve the method of achieving the decision.

Web Links

- The Mental Capacity Act 2005: www.legislation.gov.uk/ukpga/2005/9/pdfs/ukpga_20050009_en.pdf

- Making decisions: A guide for people who work in health and social care: www.gov.uk/government/uploads/system/uploads/attachment_data/file/348440/OPG603-Health-care-workers-MCA-decisions.pdf

- Mental Capacity Act 2005 – Code of Practice: www.gov.uk/government/uploads/system/uploads/attachment_data/file/497253/Mental-capacity-act-code-of-practice.pdf

- Mental Capacity – NHS Choices: www.nhs.uk/Conditions/social-care-and-support-guide/Pages/mental-capacity.aspx

7 Case-Based Discussion (Case Studies, Reflection, Action Learning)

Introduction

This chapter looks at a series of five case studies typical in paramedic practice settings. Each of these has very clear decision points which can be reflected upon and linked to the concepts discussed throughout this book. The cases are intended to be high-level examples and intentionally lack some of the details that might be seen in practice. As with all written case studies, there are no other sensory clues we usually have access to in order to enrich the context of our encounters with patients (sights, smells etc.). Despite this, the narrower dimension of written examples can be imagined in real-life practice settings, and can serve to begin prompting the use of 'decision point management' – those forks in the road which subsequent decisions rely upon.

The cases may not provide exhaustive information on every possible aspect of the scenario, and you should use any gaps you find as an opportunity to expand on the story and make further enquiry. This will provide even more opportunity to develop your skills and broaden your thinking beyond what you can see or read.

Importantly, the case studies use a 'before and after' layout, highlighting the biases and fallacies, and have some obviously intuitive outcomes which may, or may not, be correct. Remember, the most important aspect is the process you follow to achieve the answer – not the answer itself, as this may cause hindsight bias as a result. Please note – all the case studies use standard medical clerking headings/abbreviations:

- HPC: History of presenting complaint
- PMH: Previous medical (and/or surgical) history
- Allergies: Including medicines and foods
- DH: Drug history – prescribed and over the counter medicines taken
- SH: Social history (how they live)
- SE: System evaluation (sometimes called 'review of systems'). Asks the patient about symptoms organised by system, i.e. headaches
- OE: On examination – findings of physical assessments
- IMP: Impression – the working diagnosis
- Plan: Onward plan of care.

There is an appendix at the end of this chapter which contains a case study template that you could use to structure your own case studies. You can use this to assist with reflective practice cases you undertake as you develop your further decision-making skills based on encounters you have had.

Case Studies

Case Study 1: *32-year-old Female with Headache*

Background

You are working on a response car for an ambulance trust. It is a Saturday night shift at midnight and you have already attended five incidents since you started your shift at 19:00. It is your second of three night shifts. You are called to a 32-year-old female with a headache and hyperventilation. On arrival, you find the patient conscious and talking but extremely anxious. She is accompanied by her partner who is eager to get the all clear so they can continue their evening.

- HPC: Patient has been out this evening and has consumed several glasses of wine and spirits (around 8 units of alcohol), she has returned home earlier than planned due to feeling unwell. Has vomited once and since felt better. An hour later, the patient was having intercourse when the onset of headache occurred. Her partner called 999 when she started to hyperventilate and he became worried about her breathing.

- PMH: Migraine, dysmenorrhea.

- Allergies: None.

- DH: Rizatriptan, oral contraceptive pill (OCP), tranexamic acid (TXA).

- SH: Lives alone.

- SE: Patient complains of generalised headache, atypical prodrome for migraine (no aura). Denies chest pain. All other review-of-systems responses are unremarkable.

- Vital signs and clinical observations all within normal limits.

- IMP: Migraine headache and hyperventilation due to emotional factors.

- Plan: Leave at home in the care of partner.

Intuitive Responses

This presentation carries a range of risks, and leads to a decision being made entirely intuitively. Perhaps the clinician was thinking '*This must be a migraine. She has been drinking, and this has made her emotional and panicky. The hyperventilation is emotional in origin and can be managed with coaching*'. This only describes 'what' they are seeing or perceiving. There is no consideration of 'why'. Why, for example, must the hyperventilation have been caused by emotional factors? Hyperventilation may be emotional in origin, but could also be linked to sinister metabolic disturbance.

Migraine sufferers may also have intracranial bleeds, and are at higher risk of mortality due to history of primary headaches being incorrectly attributed to acute secondary headache. Coital headaches are usually self-limiting and may not have accompanying focal neurology.

Biases and Fallacies
(Review Table 4.3 in Chapter 4 to find the biases used in the example.)

- **Association bias.** Young females are prone to hyperventilation and anxiety (a picture of a young female hyperventilating is common).

- **Availability bias.** 'Emotional patient' must mean hyperventilation is emotional in origin.

What other biases and fallacies may be involved with this case?

Human Factors
- Saturday night shift (fatigue, workload, staffing levels etc.)

- Lone working

- Work intensity (number of incidents attended already)

- Tiredness

- Lack of team or other colleague to share ideas with.

What other human factors may be involved with this case?

Potential Outcome for This Patient with Poor Decision Making

The decision is made to leave the patient at home with her boyfriend. No worsening care advice is documented, and no safety netting is provided. In the early hours, the patient becomes more sleepy and so is put to bed by her boyfriend. Her intercranial pressure rises (due to an undiagnosed intracranial bleed) and causes increasing coma but this is unmonitored. The next morning, her boyfriend is unable to wake her and calls 999 who provide pre-arrival CPR instruction. An ambulance attends and crew are unable to resuscitate despite an extended period of ALS. Following application of all available interventions, the decision is taken to cease resuscitation (using appropriate decision-making process to ensure all reversible causes are addressed).

Potential Outcome for This Patient with Good Decision Making

Information Processing (Critical Analysis of Data and Information)
- History of migraine may be a fog – atypical presentation. If the patient didn't have a history of migraine, would you consider the presentation as a primary or secondary headache?

- Consideration of health history, including drug history.
- Coital headache (this onset of which may be mid-coital) – not always sinister, but sinister aspects need to be ruled out.
- Alcohol consumption may mask true level of consciousness.
- Poor historian – patient has consumed alcohol.
- Patient's boyfriend may not be worried as he wishes to continue with his evening.

Professional Insights
- I do not have the neurological assessment skills to rule out sinister pathology (*I know what I don't know*).
- I do not know enough about headaches and patients with migraine.
- I know the key differential diagnoses for headache but cannot definitively rule in/ out.

Hypotheses/Differential Diagnoses (With Positive Features – !)
- Meningitis
- Encephalitis
- Sub-arachnoid haemorrhage !
- Head injury
- Sinusitis
- Tropical illness (e.g. malaria)
- Pre-eclampsia ! (vomiting – unknown if patient is pregnant)
- Hypertensive crisis
- Migraine !
- Coital headache !
- Trigeminal neuralgia
- Glaucoma

Deductive Reasoning
- This patient may need further assessment and imaging (MRI/CT) based on the likely differential diagnoses.
- I have reached my capability line (see Chapter 5) and cannot reach a definitive diagnosis.
- I have both insufficient skills and diagnostic equipment to rule out sinister pathology.
- The only solution is to refer this patient on for further assessment.

Ethical Considerations
- Vulnerability – intoxication and in care of boyfriend (consideration should be given to the relationship status, i.e. have they just met or are they in a stable, long-term relationship?).

- Non-maleficence – prevent harm coming to patient.

- Justice – has the patient received the best care/service they deserve?

Professional Issues
Practising to scope of practice and level of competency.

The Best Outcome Using Good Decision Making Processes

This patient has a sudden onset headache and has several other issues which make it impossible to make a definitive diagnosis in this setting. A key decision as to whether to make a clinical diagnosis or refer for imaging is an intrinsic consideration of decision making in urgent and emergency care.

The patient was therefore sent to emergency department immediately and deteriorated in the ambulance en route to the hospital. On arrival, the crew were met by a team and the patient was intubated and had a CT scan. She was found to have an intracranial bleed. The plan of care was conservative treatment and she was woken on Day 3. She was discharged from hospital around a week later with no neurological deficit.

Decision Making: Assessment and Key Learning Points

Primary headaches (spontaneous in nature, such as generalised headaches) are common, and can be mistaken for secondary headaches (resulting from disease, such as a brain tumour) where the causation isn't obvious. The decision making in this case was as much about logical information processing than achieving diagnostic certainty. It was clear early on that to leave the patient at home was to take a very significant risk, and the 'before' case led to a very poor outcome. Even if the decision had been to leave the patient at home, the decision point management was very weak in the 'before' part of the case study and there was no safety netting provided. This case highlights the risks of making intuitive decisions which are influenced by associative biases, and in a setting which may introduce additional risks from human factors (i.e. fatigue). Stepping back and assessing the quality of the information and processing it in a step-wise way before testing each hypothesis will lead to an end point. That end point may not be a diagnosis, but may be the point where you reach the limit of your capability suggesting the need to refer on to hospital. The decision to say you cannot reach a diagnosis and need to refer on may affect how we feel (bruised pride, frustration). Reaching such a decision requires good levels of professional insight and self-confidence. Remembering that the patient is paramount (safety, outcomes, justice) and striving to learn from our experiences are key aspects of professional practice.

Case Study 2: *45-year-old Male with Productive Cough and Chest Pain*

Background

You are working on a double crewed ambulance with a junior colleague and have been on duty since 08:00. It been a quiet start to the shift, and at 08:17 you receive a 999 call to a 39-year-old male with a cough and chest pain.

The patient is being nagged by his partner, who is claiming he is 'putting it on' and has 'man-flu'. She was ill last week, and he didn't care when she was feeling poorly. The partner continually interrupts the encounter between you and patient.

- HPC: 5/7 history of productive cough with fever, complaining of feeling weak and suffering 'aches and pains'. Over the last 24 hours, coughing frequency has increased and he is finding it harder to clear his throat. He now has pains across his chest – described as 'muscular' and 'aching'.

- PMH: Hypertension (recent diagnosis).

- Allergies: NKDA.

- DH: ACE inhibitor.

- SH: Lives with girlfriend. Unemployed.

- SE: Denies headache or other neurological signs or symptoms. C/O increased sputum production and expectoration. C/O pain across chest – patient generalises to whole chest. Pain worse when coughing.

- OE: Hypertensive, HR 84 reg, blood glucose 5.6 mmol, temp 38.0°.

- IMP: Chest infection. Chest pain muscular in origin and caused by coughing.

- Plan: See GP later that morning for antibiotics. Discharge into care of partner.

Intuitive Responses
There are obvious signs of a chest infection, and this is probably a correct diagnosis in isolation, but remember that patients can have two acute illnesses at the same time. The crew may have been thinking along the lines of '*Clearly, the patient has a chest infection and is too young to be having a heart attack. Therefore, the chest pain can be accounted for due to the many days of constant coughing.*'

This patient should see his GP to get some antibiotics. We can leave him at home with his girlfriend.

Biases and Fallacies
(Review Table 4.3 in Chapter 4 to find the biases used in the example.)

- **Stereotyping.** Men don't tolerate minor health problems well. He probably called 999 because he was fed up with being ill.

117

- **Association bias.** Associating the productive cough, fever and chest pain with a simple diagnosis of a chest infection. The symptoms lend themselves to the diagnosis.

- **Availability bias.** Experience may lead to a recall of more middle aged men with chest infections than heart attacks. The availability and association biases have conspired to prevent effective enquiry into the true cause and nature of the chest pain.

What other biases and fallacies may be involved with this case?

Human Factors
- Distractions and interruptions – the patient's partner was being disruptive and dismissive.

- Human error – the crew missed the other cause of the chest pain.

- Poor information processing – the origin of the chest pain being muscular was not processed effectively.

- Vigilance – the crew did not diligently ensure the patient was safe and used their intuition to drive their plan.

What other human factors may be involved with this case?

Potential Outcome for This Patient with Poor Decision Making

The diagnosis given of chest infection was correct, but unrelated to this illness this patient also suffered a myocardial infarction, causing chest pain, weakness and feeling ill. The true retrosternal chest pain was masked by the muscular pains and the patient's other symptoms.

After being discharged from the paramedics' care, the patient went back to bed and rested for about 90 minutes and then rose to go to the toilet. At this point he collapsed to the floor as witnessed by his partner. She commenced CPR and called 999, receiving pre-arrival advice. A crew arrived in around 7 minutes and found the patient to have a pulse but unconscious. Upon moving to the vehicle, the patient re-arrested and was given advanced life support before gaining ROSC again. He was taken to hospital and underwent primary percutaneous coronary intervention (pPCI) to clear his occluded coronary artery. He went on to make a good recovery.

Potential Outcome for This Patient with Good Decision Making

Information Processing (Critical Analysis of Data and Information)
- Chest pain is always sinister and needs investigating (i.e. ECG).

- In the presence of other disease processes, other signs and symptoms may lose their typical nature or quality. In this case, the chest pain was masked by the muscular discomfort. The weakness and feeling of illness were attributed solely to an infection.

- There was no attempt to find out 'WHY' the patient had chest pain – they only focused on the 'WHAT'.

- Innate egocentrism – the crew believed they were correct, so thought their decision was correct without questioning it.

Professional Insights

- A potential lack of understanding of own limitations.

- Use of experience and intuition without challenge.

Hypotheses/Differential Diagnoses (With Positive Features – !)

- Acute coronary syndrome (ACS) !

- Dissecting thoracic aneurysm !

- Pericarditis/myocarditis !

- Acute congestive cardiac failure

- Pulmonary embolus !

- Acute pancreatitis

- Oesophageal rupture

- Pneumonia/Lower respiratory tract infection

Deductive reasoning

- This patient has chest pain as well as other symptoms indicative of bacterial or viral illness.

- The patient has problems I cannot visualise and so needs diagnostic tests.

- I can do some diagnostic tests, such as an ECG, but I cannot access in the community all of the tests I need.

- My working diagnosis does not rule out sinister causes for chest pain, it only rules in a chest infection.

- Therefore, this patient has undifferentiated acute chest pain and should attend hospital for repeat ECG and troponin tests.

- I have reached my capability line (see Chapter 5) and cannot reach a definitive diagnosis.

- The safe and logical decision is to convey this patient to an emergency department.

Ethical Considerations

- This patient did not get just levels of care – his needs were not addressed due to poor decision making and lack of systematic assessment.

● This case was not approached in a beneficent way. The care was not applied in the patient's best interest or on the basis of providing sufficient information for the patient to be informed about their health needs.

Professional Issues
In this case, several HCPC standards were not applied:

Identify and minimise risk

'You must refer a service user to another practitioner if the care, treatment or other services they need are beyond your scope of practice.'

'You must take all reasonable steps to reduce the risk of harm to service users, carers and colleagues as far as possible.'

'You must not do anything, or allow someone else to do anything, which could put the health or safety of a service user, carer or colleague at unacceptable risk.'

(HCPC, 2016)

There was a lack of competency in the way the patient was managed, and it could be argued that patient-centred care was not provided.

The Best Outcome Using Good Decision-Making Processes

This patient suffered a myocardial infarction about an hour prior to calling the ambulance for his worsening infective symptoms. When the ambulance crew arrived they initially focused on the chest pain, rather than the fever or other infective signs and symptoms (mindful of the risk of severe sepsis, of course). They completed an initial ECG which showed extensive ST segment elevation indicating an anterior infarct. They completed the STEMI care bundle (aspirin, nitrates, analgesia) and took the patient directly to the pPCI centre following a discussion with the team at the hospital. The clot was resolved successfully, and at no point did the patient go into cardiac arrest. After the pPCI was completed, the patient was treated for a severe chest infection alongside his cardiac aftercare.

Decision Making Assessment and Key Learning Points

While such scenarios are rare, they highlight the importance of avoiding the risk of dismissing other possibilities simply because they are rare. We have discussed previously the danger of using terms such as 'if it looks like a duck and sounds like a duck, it's probably a duck'. It could be argued that the chest infection looked and sounded like a duck, but where the two diseases (chest infection and MI) are blended, it becomes a different animal that is extremely rare and doesn't look like anything seen before.

In this case, the outcome didn't change, and the additional 90-minute delay between the initial 999 call and the eventual collapse had a minimal impact on the long-term outcome, but that is not the point. How many times are bullets dodged without our knowledge, and how many times are we correct or incorrect without knowing?

Case Study 3: *78-year-old Female Fallen with a Minor Head Injury and Taking Anticoagulant Therapy*

Background

You are on a clinical placement in a local GP practice and are asked to visit an older patient who fell at home that morning. Her sister is with her and is worried about the patient, so has called the surgery. She is a 79-year-old lady who, for her age, is in very good health. The GP knows that you have done a minor injuries course and may be able to suture the head wound and this would mean avoiding a trip to hospital. You are very keen to demonstrate your wound care competencies to the GP.

- HPC: Slipped from her chair while stretching to put something on a nearby table and hit her head on the corner of an adjacent piece of furniture. The wound on her head has bled profusely and is being managed with a tea-towel and cold compress from her sister.

- PMH: Atrial fibrillation.

- Allergies: Elastoplast.

- DH: Apixaban.

- SH: Lives with sister in an independent living setting. No other family. Has meals on wheels and attends local Age UK day centre twice a week. No social isolation noted.

- SE: The patient says she feels rather silly falling out of her chair like she did. She is worried about the blood staining the carpet. She denies headache or any other injuries, but does admit that she caught her head with quite some force. No nausea or vomiting. Able to mobilise with assistance.

- OE: Neurological exam unremarkable (cranial nerve assessment, PERRLA, Romberg's test, PNS gross movement, 'Time Up and Go'). GCS 15 – no loss of consciousness.
  5 cm laceration to vertex, bleeding freely. Large haematoma forming. All other systems/observations unremarkable or normal for patient.

- IMP: Minor fall in the home with head wound/injury. Not on warfarin, so safe to treat at home.

- Plan: Close wound with glue and steri-strips. Discharge into care of sister. Return to GP practice to update patient's notes.

Intuitive Responses
'*The main issue the GP wants me to focus on is the head wound, and this will be one of the first I have done on my own. I am anxious to demonstrate my wound care skills.*'

The paramedic in this case has discounted the fall as being sinister and is instead focusing on closing the wound, safe in the knowledge that the patient is not on warfarin and so is not at risk of a bleed. There is a presumption that the head wound is the only issue and the fall has already been deemed minor. Logically, the GP cannot possibly know the magnitude of the fall based on a request for a home visit from a relative of the patient. The lack of any wider context has further served to blinker the attending paramedic and these factors are conspiring to promote a poorly conceived intuitive response. Moreover, the well-established heuristic knowledge about the link between warfarin and head injuries in older patients, and the lack of knowledge and awareness of the novel (newer) anticoagulant drugs (NOACs) further prevents structured enquiry.

Biases and Fallacies
(Review Table 4.3 in Chapter 4 to find the biases used in the example.)

- **Confirmation bias.** Things don't cease to exist because they are ignored (or not sought) see p.73.

- **Authority bias.** Unconditional belief in what the GP said about the patient's needs.

- **Availability bias.** There was an understanding of warfarin in the context of head injury, and the absence of that medicine provided a basis to make the wrong decision because the knowledge was available (remember, we often don't know what we don't know).

What other biases and fallacies may be involved with this case?

Human Factors
- Environment – working in a new practice setting.

- Team – being on placement with a different group of staff and professional groups.

- Adverse event – the error has led to harm to the patient.

- Training – did the paramedic have sufficient training?

What other human factors may be involved with this case?

Potential Outcome for This Patient with Poor Decision Making

The patient and her sister were delighted with the care they got at the time. The patient was made comfortable in her armchair and the head wound attended to. The wound was thoroughly cleaned and closed with tissue adhesive giving a very good aesthetic result. The haematoma was still present but not getting worse and a further cold compress was applied. Oral analgesia was given, and the patient received head injury advice, including what to do if she felt ill in due course.

Later that afternoon, the patient started complaining of headache and nausea, and soon after vomited twice. Her sister noticed that she was unsteady and appeared a little confused.

At the same time, back at the GP surgery, a practice meeting was taking place to review the day's patients and home visits. When asked about the patient with the head wound, the GP said he had forgotten to mention the apixaban, and asks if the paramedic sent the patient to hospital.

The patient has started to lose consciousness and the sister calls 999. A crew arrive and take the patient to hospital where an extradural haemorrhage is noted. The patient is actively treated and recovers from the bleed and undergoes a period of rehabilitation before being discharged into a residential home, along with her sister.

The outcome for this patient is unlikely to have changed had the red flag been noted sooner, but this highlights the important nature of avoiding hindsight bias. The outcome could easily have been that the patient died quickly from a more rapidly developing bleed, and similarly a slower bleed could have led to coma during sleep that night. There are several factors relating to this case, but the most significant root cause is the lack of knowledge of common prescribing in older patients with AF. Novel anticoagulants (NOAC) are more commonly used, and have a wider range of drug names such as apixaban, dabigatran etexilate, edoxaban and rivaroxaban which need to be understood. In the past, warfarin was most commonly used and became a heuristically embedded, universally understood risk factor.

Potential Outcome for This Patient with Good Decision Making

Information Processing (Critical Analysis of Data and Information)

- Older patient fallen – why did she fall? Have all the Red Flags associated with older patients falling been considered?

- History of head injury – in older patients, the index of suspicion is far higher for brain injury, even if they are not symptomatic at the time.

- History of atrial fibrillation – why can I not see an anticoagulant on her prescription?

- Drug history reviewed but not understood – patient has AF, but anticoagulant (warfarin) not seen (see, 'Where is the bomb' in Chapter 3).

- Large developing haematoma at wound site – freely bleeding wound and a developing haematoma may suggest anticoagulant use. Recheck the medicines!

Professional Insights

- I am confident and competent to manage the wound, but may lack the insight to assess my own ability to manage wounds in older or complex patients.

- I don't know every common medicine used in primary care.

- The clinician may have thought 'My role does not require me to read all NICE guidance, some of which may not be relevant to me as I am not a prescriber. I will stick to my current knowledge.'

- Innate self-validation – 'It's true because I have always believed it'; 'Warfarin is the most common anticoagulant and the only one I know. So it may be the only one.'

Hypotheses/Differential Diagnoses (With Positive Features – !)
- Intracranial bleed secondary to trauma ! (based on risk factors)

- Skull fracture

- Minor scalp wound !

- Haematoma to scalp !

- Associated causes of fall !

Deductive Reasoning
- This patient has a large scalp wound and developing haematoma.

- She is an older patient, but essentially well.

- I can manage her wound, and should do so.

- She has suffered a blow to the head but appears neurologically intact.

- She has AF. Is she taking medicines to prevent clotting?

- There are medicines in her prescription which I don't recognise – I will check via my BNF app on my phone.

- Apixaban is an anticoagulant.

- Patients with head injuries who take anticoagulants should be seen in hospital.

- This patient has a scalp wound with a potential underlying brain injury.

Ethical Considerations
- In this case, the paramedic was very confident in how to manage the wound and became overly focused on this to the exclusion of the holistic needs of the patient. It is important to see patients as paramount, and never as a means to an end. The keenness to apply the new wound care skills could be seen as using the patient as a means to an end. It is important to approach patients based on their needs in relation to their illness or injury, rather than your own professional development and practice.

Professional Issues
Clinicians must ensure that they are competent to practise and be able to demonstrate that patients are not at risk where there is a gap in knowledge or skill.

The paramedic was unaware of the gaps in their knowledge and this led to an overall lack of competence to address the patient's needs. This in itself is not an issue as there is always the option to defer to a colleague for support, and to share decisions. This requires high levels of professional insight and the ability to assess one's own level of competency. It is far better to suffer a small dent in your pride than to harm a patient.

The Best Outcome Using Good Decision Making Processes

Using a deductive process which builds hypotheses based on critically assessed information has allowed certain factors to be tested and challenged. The key red flag relating to anticoagulant therapy has been identified and the patient is now taken to the emergency department. Early treatment is conservative, and the patient is monitored for several hours, and the same deterioration is noted in the emergency department. The scenario from here plays out in exactly the same way with the patient making a good recovery.

Decision Making Assessment and Key Learning Points

This case highlights the importance of professional insight and ensuring that any gaps in knowledge do not lead to risk of harm to patients. The deductive process, using logical arguments based on the information present, highlighted very quickly a link between the patient's condition, their acute problem, and their drug history (or apparent lack of drug history). Just because something you expect isn't there doesn't mean it doesn't exist. A patient with a freely bleeding wound and who has AF is very likely to be on an anticoagulant, and that medicine may be unfamiliar. How often do we look at a patient's list of medicines – particularly in the older patient where the list may be very long – and ignore items which are not familiar? Where a condition such as AF exists, it should draw the deductive process to resolving the likely treatment regime which the NICE guidance indicates. Remember the story from Rosenorn-Langg – airport security staff do not simply allow bags to pass through the x-ray scanner saying 'no bomb, no bomb, no bomb', instead they ask themselves 'where's the bomb?' – 'actively looking', rather than 'not seeing' (Rosenorn-Langg, 2014, p.1).

Case Study 4: *29-year-old Female with Respiratory Illness*

Background

You are working in a busy urgent care centre on a Thursday afternoon. It has been a steady day and you have seen a range of patients with minor illness and injuries throughout the day. At about 20:00 you go to the waiting room to call the next patient. The patient and her partner follow you to the consulting room. The patient is a 29-year-old female with a 5-day history of cough and fever. This is her third consultation over the past two days. She has been seen by a GP and an ambulance crew previously who have all suggested a self-limiting viral illness as originally diagnosed two days previously.

- HPC: 5-day history of worsening productive cough and increasing weakness.

- PMH: Appendicectomy aged 13. Two children, both delivered by C-Section.

- Allergies: NKDA

- DH: Oral contraceptive pill

- SH: Lives with husband and two children. Works part-time for the local authority housing team.

- SE: Complains of feeling awful. Says she 'feels like she is dying'. She appears panicky and her partner reports feeling frustrated that she is still ill and his parents are having to look after the kids. Wants to know why she is still ill and not getting better.
  Complains of feeling shivery and is coughing +++. (No further systems history reviewed as focus on viral illness affecting chest.)

- OE: HR 118, RR, 22, BP 88/45, SpO_2 94%, Temp 38.2 deg. Some adventitious chest sounds on auscultation but hard to discern as patient coughing.

- IMP: Based on previous encounters which included a GP opinion, agree that this is likely to be a viral illness which will resolve with self-care.

- Plan: Discharge with advice to use paracetamol PRN to manage fever. Aim to maintain hydration by taking clear fluids (water, dilute fruit juice) regularly.

Intuitive Responses

She has been seen by her GP who has told her what is wrong, and I am worried about looking foolish if I disagree with the GP. I do not want to contradict a senior clinician. The ambulance crew didn't find anything either presumably as she wasn't taken to hospital.

The history and symptoms still fit with the diagnosis, and the increased heart and respiratory rate are probably because she is tired and anxious. It all seems to fit and she can always come back if she doesn't get better.

Biases and Fallacies

(Review Table 4.3 in Chapter 4 to find the biases used in the example.)

- **Authority bias.** Concern about contradicting the opinion of the GP because they are a senior healthcare professional.

- **Group-think.** In this case, the paramedic, the ambulance crew and the GP all fall into a common belief that the patient had a self-limiting viral illness. Group-think can occur where information is passed around, such as in this case, and leads to a lack of challenge from each recipient.

- **Neglect of probability.** Common things happen commonly, and rare things happen rarely – but they still happen. Considering probability is important.

What other biases and fallacies may be involved with this case?

Human Factors

- Lone working – working in a setting which isn't team-based can lead to isolation, even if colleagues are present and could be called upon to help with decision making.

- Information processing – lack of critical analysis of the physiological impact of the patient's condition. The observations were clearly abnormal, but were considered in context of an existing diagnosis presumed to be correct.

- Latent error – the GP and the previously attending ambulance crew both potentially made an error in judging the patient's condition (although the patient may have presented with milder or more subtle signs earlier).

- Vigilance – the nature of work in certain clinical settings, particulary where another clinician with higher authority has already made a diagnosis, may result in a false sense of security leading to potentially missing very unwell patients.

What other human factors may be involved with this case?

Potential Outcome for This Patient with Poor Decision Making

The patient left the consulting room and walked back to the waiting room while her husband went to collect the car as she felt she couldn't walk that far. After her husband left the waiting room, the patient passes out and falls to the floor. The receptionist notices this and goes over to the patient to find her unrousable and cannot detect a pulse. She shouts for help while commencing CPR. Staff leave their consulting room to attend to the patient and an ambulance is called. The combined efforts of the ambulance paramedics and UCC staff leads to a return of spontaneous circulation, and the patient is stabilised and taken to the local hospital. Her observations are now that of a critically unwell patient, and she is carefully intubated and transferred to ITU. She requires inotropic support as well as other interventions, but sadly on day 2 it becomes clear that the overwhelming sepsis has already caused irreversible organ damage and the patient goes into cardiac arrest. Despite the best efforts of the team, the resuscitation attempt is terminated after 90 minutes.

Potential Outcome for This Patient with Good Decision Making

Information Processing (Critical Analysis of Data and Information)
- History of illness which is not improving and seems to be getting worse.

- The patient is using classic terminology associated with sepsis ('I think I am dying').

- Why did the GP think this was a viral illness, and was he correct? I should challenge his findings.

- Why did the ambulance crew also think this was a viral illness, and what made them confirm the GP's diagnosis?

- The patient's observations are outside normal ranges suggesting a systemic effect from the illness.

- Do I have enough information to make a decision? I need to expand my review of systems (SE) to include additional questions about passing urine which would have elicited that she hasn't urinated in over 8 hours. What is her NEWS score and what are the individual elements, such as the blood pressure?

Professional Insights

- Have I approached this patient correctly and not dismissed their needs because they have already seen another healthcare professional?

- Do I have the necessary skills to assess this patient in this practice setting, and does my scope of practice extend to the nature of the condition presenting?

- Am I prepared to ask for assistance in this case?

- Am I prepared to question and/or contradict a GP's diagnosis?

Hypotheses/Differential Diagnoses (With Positive Features – !)

The following are secondary to the presence of severe sepsis as the chief complaint, and may be considered as the focus of the infection:

- Upper respiratory tract infection

- Acute bronchitis !

- Pneumonia !

- Pulmonary embolism

- Bronchiectasis

- Pleurisy.

Deductive Reasoning

- This patient has an infective illness which is affecting her physiology and appears therefore to be systemic.

- This systemic infection appears to be affecting her perfusion (high NEWS score and not passing urine).

- The patient is severely septic. I will call 999 for my patient with Red Flag sepsis.

Ethical Considerations

- Non-maleficence – it is vital to prevent harm coming to the patient, and this extends to ensuring diseases are identified and their progression minimised.

- Justice – the patient has had three healthcare encounters and yet has not been given the correct care.

Professional Issues

In this case, there was a lack of appreciation of the needs of the patient, and the lack of structured decision making placed the patient in jeopardy. It is reasonable to consider the possibility that had the patient self-presented to the urgent care centre without first seeing other healthcare professionals/services, a more thorough assessment may have taken place. From a professional regulation perspective, this case has features which may be contrary to the published standards, such as:

> '*be able to assess a professional situation, determine the nature and severity of the problem and call upon the required knowledge and experience to deal with the problem*'

(HCPC, 2014)

The Best Outcome Using Good Decision Making Processes

The patient presented to the urgent care centre and was called through by the paramedic. When the patient mentioned the previous diagnosis given by the GP, and which was subsequently confirmed by the ambulance crew, the paramedic makes it clear to the patient that they would assess her thoroughly and objectively and that she was correct to attend this afternoon. It quickly becomes apparent that despite the vital signs and the previous diagnosis given, this patient has severe sepsis. She is gravely ill, but is currently compensating well. The patient is screened using the Trust's sepsis protocol and a 999 call is made straightaway. An ambulance arrives within 10 minutes and the patient receives IV fluids and is taken to hospital as a priority call using blue lights and sirens. On arrival at ED she receives IV antibiotics and is transferred to ITU. She remained unstable for the first 24 hours but eventually improves and recovers. She is discharged several weeks later and has damage to her kidneys, but is grateful to be alive. The ITU consultant stated upon her discharge how close to death she had been at one point.

Decision Making Assessment and Key Learning Points

On some occasions, logical deduction drives the type of management rather than the final diagnosis. This patient's overall condition raised alarm in the paramedic in the 'best outcome' section, and this intuition appropriately drove hypotheses which in turn led to screening the patient against known parameters (the sepsis protocol). While a respiratory illness was most likely, the final diagnosis was not made. In the case of severe sepsis, it is more important to resuscitate than to find the type or focus of the infection, as antibiotic therapy may be given empirically rather than waiting for microbiology tests to confirm the bug causing the infection. More importantly is the need to ensure that a decision is made, and that previous decisions are not adopted without your own enquiry. This case shows how easy it can be to write off a patient with very marked features of disease processes – both in terms of signs and symptoms, and changes to their physiology – just because another clinician has given a diagnosis. If the paramedic had not been aware of the previous visits to the GP or the 999 call that the ambulance crew attended, would they have thought differently?

Case Study 5: *36-year-old Female with Abdominal Pain*

Background

You are working on a response car on Sunday night shift in early summer. At about midnight, you receive a 999 call to a female complaining of abdominal pain. The call has come from the NHS111 service which has assessed the call as needing an ambulance response due to the responses to the triage questions.

On arrival, you are taken to the patient who is lying on the sofa watching television. She complains of lower abdominal discomfort.

- HPC: 3/7 history of 'gripey' pain. Non-radiating. No fever. Patient states she is 'fed up with the pain' and wants to feel better.

- PMH: Two recent terminations of pregnancy (both in the last 12 months). Learning disability. Mild asthma.

- Allergies: NKDA.

- DH: None.

- SH: Lives with partner. Works part-time in local shop. Has a support worker who assists with certain aspects of her life.

- SE: Complains of pain across lower abdomen. Bowels open normally and no concerns regarding 'water works'.
  Nauseated. Vomited x 1. No diarrhoea.
  Denies headache, chest pain and breathing problems. All other systems reviewed are negative to symptoms.

- Denies pregnancy and denies sexual activity.

- OE: HR 105, RR 16, BP 105/65, SaO₂ 98%, Pain score 6/10
  Abdomen soft. Tender to light palpation in LLQ and RLQ quadrants.

- IMP: Abdominal pain ?cause in a patient of childbearing age with a recent history of termination of pregnancy.

- Plan: Seek consent to undertake urinalysis and confirm findings (bHCG +ve. Blood ++).

Intuitive Responses

This patient has abdominal pain, and I know that if I try for a diagnosis I am likely to be wrong. (According to Simon et al., 2005, 50% of initial diagnoses for abdominal pain are wrong.) The patient may not fully understand the questions I am asking about being pregnant or the true meaning of sexual activity due to her learning disability. I am also concerned about her potential vulnerability and the history of multiple terminations.

I am going ask the patient for a urine sample to test for a potential urinary tract infection, but also to ensure she is not pregnant.

Biases and Fallacies
(Review Table 4.3 in Chapter 4 to find the biases used in the example.)

False causality. Assumption that a patient with learning disability is unaware of her own sexual health. She may be aware but unable to express this in terms understood by those not known to the patient.

Conjunction. Linking the cause of a potential unknown pregnancy to the patient's competency. The cause of the abdominal pain is an undetected ectopic pregnancy, not the patient's learning disability.

Feature-positive effect. This has been avoided in this case. Commonly, things that cannot be seen are ignored, and in this case the potential issue has been identified and searched for.

What other biases and fallacies may be involved with this case?

Human Factors
- Skills gap – lack of knowledge of learning disabilities.

- Communication – loss of opportunity to ask the patient to express herself in her own terms.

What other human factors may be involved with this case?

Actual Outcome for This Patient with Poor Decision Making

The decision making in this case was technically very good. The possibility of being unaware of a pregnancy and linking this to the cause of abdominal pain was well founded through logical thought process and critical analysis of the information. Linked to this was the insight into the limitations of one's own practice.

There are some limitations with the approach to the patient's learning disability, and this has skewed the decision-making process due to biases and a lack of appreciation of the patient's functional ability.

Overall, this case describes good decision-making process and a good outcome. This scenario could have turned out very differently had the paramedic not applied a logical approach to the problem and simply trusted the patient. The differential diagnoses for a young female who is not pregnant have very few, if any, immediately sinister pathologies, and therefore missing the pregnancy (which in this case was ectopic) would represent a potentially life-threatening problem.

Actual Outcome for This Patient with Good Decision Making

Information Processing (Critical Analysis of Data and Information)
- History of abdominal pain – clinical diagnoses may be wrong in 50% of cases. Usually need follow up in secondary care. Where sinister conditions can be ruled out, follow up may be done more routinely.

- Learning disability – the patient functions well with minimal support in the community, but may not be able to express themselves, and this makes their history harder to elicit.

- Previous history of elective termination of pregnancy – what were the circumstances, and do these represent a Safeguarding issue? (Consider referral.)

- Abdomen tender.

- Pregnancy test positive.

- Reliability of urinalysis.

Professional Insights
- I am not confident to rule out sinister pathology in a patient with a learning disability as I do not understand it sufficiently.

- I may not be able to communicate as effectively with this patient and I need to be careful in how I ask them to undertake a urine test to check for pregnancy.

Hypotheses/Differential Diagnoses (With Positive Features – !)
- Appendicitis !

- Pelvic inflammatory disease !

- Pregnancy !

- Ectopic pregnancy !

- Hernia !

- Diverticulitis !

- Bowel obstruction !

- UTI

- Pyelonephritis

- Ruptured ovarian cyst !

- Bowel perforation

- Inflammatory bowel disease !

Deductive Reasoning
- This patient has a history of abdominal pain.

- Abdominal pain is very challenging to definitively diagnose in the community unless sinister features can be excluded.

- The patient denies sexual activity, but has clearly been sexually active in the past (gravida 2, para 0).

- I need to carry out urinalysis to rule out pregnancy as a cause.

- Pregnancy test (bHCG) positive.

- Pain in early pregnancy carries risk of ectopic presentation.

- I cannot manage this presentation in this setting.

- This patient needs to go to hospital urgently.

Ethical Considerations
- This patient is potentially vulnerable and should be subject to a Safeguarding referral.

Professional Issues
This case highlights the importance of professional insight and a willingness to determine one's own limitations, but this does not need to diminish good decision making. Having weaknesses in certain areas (such as in this case with learning disabilities) drives learning and reflection, and does not infer a lack of wider competency. Paramedics are arguably best described against the literature as 'generalists/extended generalists' (Benner, 1984) and may not be exposed to patients such as this on a regular basis.

The Best Outcome Using Good Decision Making Processes

The patient attended the emergency department at the local hospital and underwent further blood and urine tests to confirm pregnancy. An ultrasound scan showed an empty uterus, helping confirm that the pregnancy was ectopic and at risk of rupture. The patient went to theatre later that day and went on to make a full recovery. She went home a few days later and met with her support worker and social worker to ensure that the relationship she is in is appropriate and to offer specific support relating to her sexual health.

Decision Making Assessment and Key Learning Points

Relying on logical decision making can help overcome any gaps by applying the same processes consistently and challenging information critically rather than simply accepting what you hear. Abdominal pain in females of childbearing age carries the same physical health risks for any patient suffering with it regardless of any other circumstance, and introducing a learning disability provides an example of how the principles of good decision making can overcome additional complexities by processing the data and turning the 'what?' into 'why?' Imagine if the paramedic had accepted the patient's denial of sexual activity as a 'what' and therefore treated it as a fact – this would have been a fork in the road early on in the encounter which would inform all other decisions and is therefore critical.

Think back to the bagatelle board example in Chapter 3 and consider the focus of possible differential diagnoses in the absence of pregnancy related issues. It's vital to ask yourself 'why' did she give the answer she gave and challenge yourself to ensure that you understood it in the way the patient intended. Patients may use euphemisms or other colloquialisms to describe things to avoid embarrassment, or because it was a term used in childhood. We should ensure that we learn to receive information rather than expect patients to present it in our preferred way.

There are references in this book which encourage a level of healthy scepticism when analysing data, and this must be balanced against ensuring we build and maintain trust between us and our patient, but sometimes patients may not be able or willing to give the answer we expect for a variety of reasons.

Appendix

Case Study Template

Patient name:			
Background:			
Vital Signs			RED FLAGS
Physical examination			RED FLAGS
Other observations			RED FLAGS
Intuitive Responses	WHAT?	WHY?	RED FLAGS
Potential Biases		Effects of biases	
Fallacies		Effects of fallacies	
Human Factors		Effects	

Deductive Reasoning		
Ethical Considerations	Positive	Negative
Professional Issues	Positive	Negative
Hypotheses/Differential Diagnoses		

EVALUATION Critical Analysis of Data and Information	
What went well?	What could have gone better?
Learning points	
Professional insights	

Glossary

Absolutism   Application of an idea or principle to the exclusion of other considerations.

Action-biased   Human tend to prefer doing something rather than nothing, even where they are not trained to do something, or the action is counterproductive. Action bias in healthcare may be seen where the clinician perceives a lack of time to think before acting, or isn't aware they should think before acting.

Acuity   Acuteness or sharpness. In healthcare it usually refers to the severity of a patient's condition (for example, 'polytrauma patients are high acuity').

Acumen   Astuteness. Often used in reference to growing an ability or knowledge. In this book, we refer to building your decision-making acumen.

Aetiology   The cause, or nature of cause, of a disease. For example, the link between obesity and diabetes.

Affect heuristics   Intuitive responses able to be completed competently but influenced by emotion, such as when someone reacts to a car backfiring by running away prior to realising it isn't gunfire. The turning and running is the heuristic ability and the emotion (fear) provides the affect.

Agency   The capacity to act. Often used interchangeably with autonomy, and is linked closely with biomedical ethics.

Allied Health Professionals   The group of healthcare professionals led by the Chief Allied Health Professions Office within NHS England. Distinct from medicine and nursing.

Anthropometrics   Designing something with the end user's comfort in mind. For example, ensuring a worktop is at the correct height to prevent stooping.

Authority bias   Being influenced by someone by dint of their rank or seniority, rather than being right or wrong.

Autonomy   Able to be self-governing. Different to agency, but often used interchangeably. Autonomy is more the right to self-determination whereas agency is the ability or capacity to act.

Base-rate neglect   Ignoring the baseline information upon which context is derived. For example, believing that all immigrants are criminals because 75% of crimes in an area were carried out by immigrants, regardless of the number of immigrants in the area or how many crimes were carried out by the same people. The baseline is the immigrant population and the crime statistics should be considered in light of the baseline (base rate) rather than in isolation.

Beneficence   An act that is done for a patient's benefit. Beneficent acts may prevent harm or further harm, and/or can be used to improve the patient's situation.

bHCG test   Beta Human Gonadotrophic Hormone blood or urine test. The bHCG hormone is produced only in pregnancy and its presence indicates the patient is pregnant. May return a false positive, but rarely a false negative unless tested too early in pregnancy.

Biomedical ethics   Refers to the examination of the ethics of all biomedical research, medicine, and healthcare.

Cognition   Mental action or process of acquiring knowledge and understanding. Using your brain to provide an answer or solution – working something out; deducing.

Cognitive continuum   The gradient between scientific enquiry and pure intuition relating to decision making.

Cognitive dissonance   The discomfort felt when a person has two competing beliefs regarding a particular issue or concept, leading to contradiction and internal conflict – particularly when considering new evidence.

Cognitive tasks   Tasks needing cognitive input (thoughts, considerations, judgements). Mental arithmetic for example.

Comorbidity   Diseases which a patient has or acquires on top of an existing disease. For instance, if a patient with heart failure then develops dementia, the dementia is the comorbidity.

Confirmation bias   Using information or evidence to support pre-existing beliefs or decisions – often selectively (i.e. a normal ECG in the patient with chest pain does not in isolation support the conclusion that the patient is not having a heart attack).

Conformism   A conformist tends to follow the prevailing culture, beliefs or standards and may not question or challenge.

Conjunction bias   Conjoining concepts in a convenient way – leaping to conclusions.

Demography   Data on the composition of populations, including births, deaths, income, epidemiology.

Deontological ethics   Duty or obligation. Judgements of actions based on normative rules. For instance, the reasonable assumption, as well as prevailing laws, that killing people is morally wrong.

Diagnostic reasoning   Often referred to as 'clinical decision making', links the specific ability to use the tools described in this book to make a diagnosis.

Encephalitis   Swelling of the brain.

Encephalopathy   Diseases which affect brain functioning, such as infections or injuries.

Epidemiology   The study of disease prevalence among populations, for example, coronary heart disease in different towns and cities in a country. May be linked to demography and levels of deprivation.

Epistemology   The theory of knowledge and its acquisition.

Ergonomics   Designing things to be efficient and comfortable.

Ethnocentrism   The belief that one's own group or culture is superior to other groups.

Experiential   A word that describes knowledge based on experience or observation. Often used to imply superiority of knowledge and skills. Experience should be consolidated and reflected upon.

False causality bias   The incorrect assumption that sequential events are linked. In the decision-making context, an example is assuming that a 3-day history of coughing is the cause of the patient's chest pain, when in fact the patient is having a heart attack. This bias features heavily when considering purely intuitive decision making.

Group-think   The situation where a group of people create a consensus which other members of the group may fail to challenge, even if the consensus is wrong. People tend to not speak out rather than risk being wrong, or being seen as an outsider or opposed to the view of the group.

HCPC   The Health and Care Professions Council, the regulator for 14 health and social care professions. The HCPC is overseen by the PSA (Professional Standards Authority) which also oversees the General Medical Council (GMC) and the Nursing and Midwifery Council (NMC).

HEMS   Helicopter Emergency Medical Service. Air ambulance services which are commonly physician-led, but may also be paramedic-led.

Hermeneutics   The theory and methodology of text interpretation, especially the interpretation of biblical texts, wisdom literature, and philosophical texts. Hermeneutics was initially applied to the interpretation, or exegesis, of scripture.

Hernia   Where an organ protrudes through the wall of the cavity containing it. The most common hernias are inguinal, where a small length of intestine protrudes through the inguinal canal.

Heuristics   Obtaining knowledge through experimentation (trial and error) leading to tacit understanding sufficient to solve most issues relating to the subject.

Holistic   Treatment of the 'whole person' rather than just the disease, and includes mental/psychological and social needs and considerations.

Human factors   The influence environments and systems have on human beings, and which can lead to errors or other issues.

Hypothesis   An idea put forward for testing deductively. Differential diagnoses are hypotheses in the healthcare setting.

Hypothetico-deduction   A process of scientific enquiry used to test hypotheses in order to reach the correct answer.

Ideation   The formation of ideas. In healthcare, it may be used in the context of mental health crises where a patient expresses 'suicidal ideation' – suggesting that they are forming ideas about possible ways to end their life.

Illusory superiority   An overestimation of one's ability. There are lots of examples in healthcare where this can lead to risk of harm to patients. An example in life in general may be experienced when you hear someone say 'hold my beer'!

Ischaemic bowel   Loss of blood supply to the bowel, leading to loss of function and death of the section of bowel. May lead to peritonitis and can be fatal.

Justice   In relation to biomedical ethics, justice is defined as the patient receiving what is minimally reasonable or should be expected in terms of care, treatment and level of service.

Known knowns   That which you are confident that you know to the point where you can demonstrate the knowledge to yourself or others.

Known unknowns   Subjects for which you know you do not have sufficient knowledge. Clinicians who can express their known unknowns are demonstrating good levels of insight into their own practice and are less prone to illusory superiority.

Latent error   Contributory factors, or smaller cumulative errors which can lead to larger scale issues, but which are often overlooked.

Learning culture / no blame culture   Organisations which seek to learn from untoward incidents and errors are said to have a 'no blame' and/or 'learning culture'. Assigning blame rarely addresses the true root cause of an error or incident, and sharing learning is vital to ensure incidents are not repeated. This can only happen where clinicians feel sufficiently safe to report errors and incidents.

Loss aversion   The preference to avoid losing than trying to achieve gain. It is preferable not to lose a £10 note than to find a £10 pound note.

Mental capacity   An individuals' ability to make their own choices and decisions.

Morbidity   The condition of being diseased. Having a disease or injury, or a condition considered pathological (i.e. morbid obesity – the obesity is such that it is affecting the patient's normal function as though they were sick or injured).

Multi-morbidity   The presence of two or more major diseases at the same time. Different from comorbidity in that there is more than one primary condition being treated actively.

Murphy's Sign   A physical assessment technique used to identify pain in the gall bladder.

Myocardial infarction   Blockage of a coronary artery impairing blood flow to the heart muscle leading to ischaemia and loss of function. Can lead to cardiac arrest and death.

Non-maleficence   'Do no harm'. Ensuring that the treatment being given will not cause greater discomfort or risk to the patient without due consideration of the benefits.

Obturator test   A physical assessment technique which elicits irritation of the *obturator internus* muscle and helps with the diagnosis of appendicitis.

Polypharmacy   The prescribing of four or more medicines to patients aged over 65. Polypharmacy is associated with other risks to the patient, such as increased risk of falling.

Positivism   Only recognising that which can be proven scientifically, and rejects concepts such as theism and metaphysics.

Post-positivism   The acceptance that what we see may be wrong and that evidence may be updated.

Psoas sign   A physical assessment technique which elicits irritation to the iliopsoas group of hip flexor muscles in the abdomen. It helps identify the location of the appendix relative to the caecum.

Quasi-rationality   Quasi means something resembling another concept. The term Rationality simply means that something was done for, or with, reason.

Right iliac fossa   A depression in the right iliac region of the abdomen where pain or tenderness may be elicited in the presence of appendicitis commonly.

ROSC   Return of Spontaneous Circulation. Successfully restarting a patient's heart who has been in cardiac arrest sufficient for the patient's circulation to support itself.

Rote-learning   Learning which is achieved through habitual or repetitive study, and occasionally without the underpinning understanding. For example, learning times tables at school without learning why or how to make calculation easier.

Rovsing's test   A physical assessment technique used to assist in the diagnosis of appendicitis. It involves palpating the left lower quadrant in order to elicit pain in the right lower quadrant.

Shared decision making   Decision making that usually takes place between patient and clinician during care planning or other decision making about treatment. It can also refer to the collaborative decision making between clinicians used to assist clinicians working in isolation.

Sociocentricity   Focus on one's own social group or culture. Parochialism.

Socratic Paradox   This paradox provides the origin of the four statements relating to knowledge: I know what I know; I know what I don't know; I don't know what I know; and I don't know what I don't know.

Suturing   Closure of a wound using sutures (stitches).

System 1 thinking   Fast, intuitive thinking using the 'old' part of our brain.

System 2 thinking   Slow, deliberate thinking using the 'newer' parts of our brain.

Bibliography

See also individual chapter bibliographies

Air Line Pilots' Association (1977) *Air Accident Report (Tenerife Air Disaster).* Available: http://project-tenerife.com/engels/PDF/alpa.pdf. Last accessed February 2017.

Agan, R.D. (1987) Intuitive knowing as a dimension of nursing. *Advances in Nursing Science*, 10(1): 63–70.

Allied Health Professions Federation (2016) *Member Organisations.* Available: http://www.ahpf.org.uk/member_organisations.htm. Last accessed September 2016.

Ashforth, B.E., Harrison, S.H. and Corley, K.G. (2008) *Identification in Organizations: An Examination of Four Fundamental Questions*, p.334. Available at: http://leeds-faculty.colorado.edu/dahe7472/Journal%20of%20Management-2008-Ashforth-325-74.pdf. Last accessed February 2017.

Association of Ambulance Chief Executives (AACE) (2011). *Taking Healthcare to the Patient 2: A review of 6 years' progress and recommendations for the future.* London: AACE.

Babbage, C. (1864) *Passages from the Life of a Philosopher.* London: Longman and Co. p.67.

Baron, J. (2006) *Against Bioethics.* Cambridge, MA: MIT Press.

Bastick, T. (1982) *How We Think and Act.* New York: John Wiley.

Beauchamp, T.L. and Childress, J.F. (2001) *Principles of Biomedical Ethics*, 5th ed. Oxford: Oxford University Press.

Benner, P. (1984) *From Novice to Expert.* Menlo Park, CA: Addison-Wesley.

Benner, P. and Tanner, C. (1987) Clinical judgement: how expert nurses use intuition. *American Journal of Nursing*, 87(1): 23–34.

Bonner, A. (2003) Recognition of expertise: an important concept in the acquisition of nephrology nursing expertise. *Nursing and Health Sciences*, 5(2): 123–31.

Bordage, G. (1999) Why did I miss the diagnosis? Some cognitive explanations and educational implications. *Academic Medicine*, 74(10): S138–42.

Cambridge Dictionary (2017). Available at: http://dictionary.cambridge.org/dictionary/english. Last accessed February 2017.

Bibliography

Carnevali, D.L., Mitchell, P.H., Woods, N.F. and Tanner, C.A. (1984) *Diagnostic Reasoning in Nursing*. Philadelphia: Lippincott.

Carper, B. (1978) Fundamental ways of knowing in nursing. *Advances in Nursing Science*, 1(1): 13–23.

Charlin, B., Tardif, J. and Boshuizen, H.P.A. (2000) Scripts and medical diagnostic knowledge: theory and applications for clinical reasoning instruction and research. *Academic Medicine*, 75(2): 182–90.

Christensen, M. and Hewitt-Taylor, J. (2006) From expert to tasks, expert nursing practice redefined? *Issues in Clinical Nursing*, 15(12): 1531–9.

Cianfrani, K.L. (1984) The influence of amounts and relevance of data on identifying health problems. In Kim, M.J., McFarland, G.K. and McLane, A.M. (eds) *Classifications of Nursing Diagnoses: Proceedings of the Fifth National Conference*. St Louis: Mosby.

Cioffi, J. (1997 Heuristics, servants to intuition, in clinical decision making. *Journal of Advanced Nursing*, 26: 203–8.

Cioffi, J. (2002 What are clinical judgements? In Thompson, C. and Dowding, D. (eds) *Clinical Decision Making and Judgement in Nursing*. Edinburgh: Churchill Livingstone.

Clack, G. (2009) Decision making in nursing practice: a case review. *Paediatric Nursing*, 21(5): 24–7.

Clinical Human Factors Group (CHFG) (2015) *Human Factors in Healthcare: Common Terms*. Available: http://chfg.org/what-are-clinical-human-factors. Last accessed July 2016.

College of Paramedics (2015) *Paramedic Career Framework*, 3rd ed. Available: www.collegeofparamedics.co.uk/downloads/Post-Reg_Career_Framework_3rd_Edition.pdf. Last accessed July 2016.

College of Paramedics (2017) *Home Page*. Available: www.collegeofparamedics.co.uk/. Last accessed July 2016.

Department for Communities and Local Government (DCLG) (2015) *The English Indices of Deprivation 2015*. Available: www.gov.uk/government/uploads/system/uploads/attachment_data/file/465791/English_Indices_of_Deprivation_2015_-_Statistical_Release.pdf. Last accessed September 2016.

Department for Transport (DoT) (2014) *Annual Road Fatalities*. Available: www.gov.uk/government/publications/annual-road-fatalities. Last accessed July 2016.

Department of Health (DH) (2005) *Taking Healthcare to the Patient: Transforming NHS Ambulance Services.* London: Department of Health.

Department of Health (2012). *Long Term Conditions Compendium of Information*, 3rd ed. London: Department of Health: p.3.

Department of Health (2015) *2010 to 2015 Government Policy: Long Term Health Conditions.* Available: www.gov.uk/government/publications/2010-to-2015-government-policy-long-term-health-conditions/2010-to-2015-government-policy-long-term-health-conditions. Last accessed October 2016.

Dobelli, R. (2013). *The Art of Thinking Clearly.* London: Spectre.

Dowding, D., Spilsbury, K.,Thompson, C., Brownlow, R. and Pattenden, J. (2009) The decision making of heart failure specialist nurses in clinical practice. *Journal of Clinical Nursing*, 18: 1313–24.

Dowie, J. and Elstein, A. (1988) *Professional Judgement: A Reader in Clinical Decision Making.* Cambridge: Cambridge University Press.

Dreyfus, H.L. and Dreyfus, S. (1980) *A Five-Stage Model of the Mental Activities Involved in Direct Skill Acquisition.* Unpublished Study, University of California, Berkeley, San Francisco, CA.

Dunning, D. and Kruger, J. (1999) Unskilled and unaware of it: how difficulties in recognizing one's own incompetence lead to inflated self-assessments. *Journal of Personality and Social Psychology*, 77(6): 1121–34.

Easen, P. and Wilcockson, J. (1996) Intuition and rational decision-making in professional thinking: a false dichotomy. *Journal of Advanced Nursing*, 24: 667–73.

Elstein, A.S. and Schwarz, A. (2002) Clinical problem solving and diagnostic decision making: selective review of the cognitive literature. *British Medical Journal*, 423(7339): 729–32.

Elstein, A.S., Shulman, L.S. and Sprafka, S.A. (1978) *Medical Problem Solving: An Analysis of Clinical Reasoning.* Cambridge, MA: Harvard University Press.

English, I. (1993) Intuition as a function of the expert nurse: a critique of Benner's Novice to Expert model. *Journal of Advanced Nursing*, 18: 387–93.

Eraut, M. (1994) *Developing Professional Knowledge and Competence.* London: The Falmer Press.

Gallagher, A., Vyvyan, E., Juniper, J., Snook, V., Horsfield, C., Collen, A. and Rutland, S. (2016) Consensus towards understanding and sustaining professionalism in paramedic practice. *British Paramedic Journal*, 1(2): 1–8.

Gambrill, E. (2012) *Critical Thinking in Clinical Practice*, 3rd ed. Hoboken, USA: John Wiley.

Gilhooly, K.S. (1990) Cognitive psychology and medical diagnosis. *Applied Cognitive Psychology*, 4: 534–52.

Grant, J. and Marsden, P. (1987) The structure of memorized knowledge in students and clinicians: an explanation for diagnostic expertise. *Medical Education*, 21: 92.

Greenhalgh, T. and Hurwitz, B. (1998) *Narrative Based Medicine: Dialogue and Discourse in Clinical Practice*. London: BMJ Books.

Griffiths, B. (1978) Some comments on McDonalds paper. *Educational Studies in Mathematics*, 9: 87.

Hamers, J.P.H., Huijer Abu Saad, H. and Halfens, R.J.G. (1994). Diagnostic process and decision making in nursing: a literature review. *Journal of Professional Nursing*, 10(3): 154–63.

Hamm, R. (1988) Clinical intuition and clinical analysis: expertise and the cognitive continuum. In Dowie, J. and Eisten, A. (eds) *Professional Judgement: A Reader in Clinical Decision Making*. Cambridge: Cambridge University Press.

Hammond, K.R. (1981) *Principles of Organization in Intuitive and Analytical Cognition (Report 231)*. Boulder, CO: Center for Research on Judgement and Policy, University of Colorado.

Hammond, K.R. (1996) *Human Judgement and Social Policy: Irreducible Uncertainty, Inevitable Error, Unavoidable Injustice*. New York: Oxford University Press.

Haney, C., Banks, W.C. and Zimbardo, P.G. (1973) A study of prisoners and guards in a simulated prison. *Naval Research Review*, 30: 4–17.

Health and Care Professions Council (HCPC) (2012) *Confidentiality - guidance for registrants*. Available: https://www.hcpc-uk.org/resources/guidance/confidentiality---guidance-for-registrants/. Last accessed October 2016.

Health and Care Professions Council (HCPC) (2014) *Standard of Proficiency: Paramedics*. Available: https://www.hcpc-uk.org/standards/standards-of-proficiency/paramedics/. Last accessed October 2016.

Health and Care Professions Council (HCPC) (2015) *Indicative Sanctions Policy*. Available: https://www.hcpts-uk.org/legislation/panellegislation/indicative-sanctions-policy/. Last accessed April 2017.

Health and Care Professions Council (HCPC) (2016) *Standards of Conduct, Performance and Ethics.* Available: https://www.hcpc-uk.org/standards/standards-of-conduct-performance-and-ethics/. Last accessed May 2016.

Hicks, C. (1998) Barriers to evidence based care in nursing: historical legacies and conflicting cultures. *Health Services Management Research*, 11: 137–47.

Higgs, J., Jones, M.A., Loftus, S. and Christensen, N. (2008) *Clinical Reasoning in the Health Professions*, 3rd ed. Oxford: Elsevier.

Hope, T. (2004) *Medical Ethics: A Very Short Introduction.* Oxford: Oxford University Press.

Huxley, A. (1927) *Proper Studies.* London: Chatto and Windus.

Ibarra, H. (1999) *Provisional Selves: Experimenting with Image and Identity in Professional Adaptation.* Available: http://web.mit.edu/curhan/www/docs/Articles/15341_Readings/Self-presentation_Impression_Formation/Ibarra_1999_Provisional_selves.pdf. Last accessed October 2016.

Kahneman, D. (2011) *Thinking Fast and Slow.* London: Penguin.

Kant, Immanuel, *trans.* Jonathan Bennett (2008) *Grounding for the Metaphysics of Morals,* 3rd ed. Indianapolis: Hackett, p.30.

King, I. and Clark, J.M. (2002) Intuition and the development of expertise in surgical ward and intensive care nurses. *Journal of Advanced Nursing*, 37(4): 322–9.

Kings Fund (2016) *Long Term Conditions and Multi-morbidity.* Available: www.kingsfund.org.uk/time-to-think-differently/trends/disease-and-disability/long-term-conditions-multi-morbidity. Last accessed November 2016.

Klein, G.A., Orasanu, J.M. and Calderwood, R. (1993). *Decision Making in Action: Models and Methods.* Norwood, NJ: Ablex.

Korn, Denis (2016) *Barriers to Critical Thinking.* Available at: http://learntoprepare.com/2011/06/barriers-to-critical-thinking/. Last accessed April 2016.

Kremer, M.J., Faut-Callahan, M. and Hicks, F.D. (2002) A study of clinical decision making by certified registered nurse anesthetists. *American Association of Nurse Anesthetists Journal*, 70(5): 391–7.

Lamond, D. and Thompson, C. (2000) Intuition and analysis in decision making and choice. *Journal of Nursing Scholarship*, 32(3): 411–14.

Larkin, J., McDermott, J., Simon, O.P. and Simon, H.A. (1980) Expert and novice performance in solving physics problems. *Science*, 208(4450): 1335–42.

Lovegrove, M. and Davis, J. (2013) *Paramedic Evidence Based Education Project (PEEP)*. Bridgwater: College of Paramedics.

Manias, E. and Street, A. (2001) Nurses and doctors communicating through medication order charts in critical care. *Australian Critical Care*, 14(1): 17–23.

Muir, N. (2004) Clinical decision making: theory and practice. *Nursing Standard*, 18(36): 47–52.

Murdoch, I. (1971) *The Sovereignty of Good*. London: Routledge.

National Institute for Health and Care Excellence (NICE) (2016) *Improving Health and Social Care Through Evidence-based Guidance*. Available: www.nice.org.uk/. Last accessed May 2016.

NHS Digital (2014) *National Statistics Ambulance Services, England 2013–14*. Available: http://content.digital.nhs.uk/catalogue/PUB14601. Last accessed April 2017.

NHS England (2013) *Transforming Urgent and Emergency Care Services in England. Urgent and Emergency Care Review, End of Phase 1 Report*. Available: www.nhs.uk/NHSEngland/keogh-review/Documents/UECR.Ph1Report.FV.pdf. Last accessed July 2016.

NHS England. (2014a) *The 6Cs*. Available: https://www.healthcareers.nhs.uk/about/working-health/6cs. Last accessed November 2016.

NHS England (2014b) *The Five Year Forward View*. Available: www.england.nhs.uk/wp-content/uploads/2014/10/5yfv-web.pdf. Last accessed November 2016.

NHS England (2016) *Confidentiality Policy*. Available: https://www.england.nhs.uk/publication/confidentiality-policy/. Last accessed April 2017.

Noddings, N. and Shore, P.J. (1984) *Awakening the Inner Eye: Intuition in Education*. London: Teachers College Press.

Office for National Statistics (ONS) (2015) *Population Projections*. Available: www.ons.gov.uk/peoplepopulationandcommunity/populationandmigration/populationprojections. Last accessed July 2016.

Offredy, M. (1998) The application of decision making concepts by nurse practitioners in primary care. *Journal of Advanced Nursing*, 40: 988–1000.

Oxford English Dictionary (OED) (2013) Available: http://www.oed.com/. Last accessed July 2016.

Paris Jr, J.F. (2014). *Lessons from Mount Stupid*. Available: https://josephparis.me/my-articles/lessons-from-mt-stupid/. Last accessed May 2016.

Patel, V.L. and Groen, G.J. (1986) Knowledge based solution strategies in medical reasoning. *Cognitive Science*, 10: 91–116.

Paul, R. and Elder, L. (2001) *The Miniature Guide to Critical Thinking: Concepts and Tools*. Tomales: Foundation for Critical Thinking.

Philips, L. and Rempushki, V. (1985) A decision making model for diagnosing and intervening in elder abuse and neglect. *Nursing Research*, 34(3): 134–9.

Pyles, S. and Stern, P. (1983) Discovery of nursing gestalt in critical care nursing: the importance of the Grey Gorilla Syndrome image. *Journal of Nursing Scholarship*, XV(2): 51–2.

Radwin, L.E. (1990) Research on diagnostic reasoning in nursing. *Nursing Diagnosis*, 1(2): 70–77.

Rew, L. (1986) Intuition concept analysis of a group phenomenon. *Advances in Nursing Science*, 8(2): 21–8.

Rimoldi, H. (1988) Diagnosing the diagnostic process. *Medical Education*, 22(4): 270–78.

Rosenorn-Lanng, D. (2014) *Human Factors in Healthcare*. Oxford: Oxford University Press.

Runzheimer, J. and Johnson Larsen, L. (2011) *Medical Ethics for Dummies*. Hoboken: Wiley.

Schaeffer, J. (1974) The interrelatedness of decision making and the nursing process. *American Journal of Nursing*, 74(10): 1852–5.

Schon, D. (1983) *The Reflective Practitioner: How Professionals Think in Action*. London: Temple Smith.

Simon, C., Everitt, H. and Kendrick, T. (2005) *Oxford Handbook of General Practice*. Oxford: Oxford University Press.

Simons, D. (2010) *The Monkey Business Illusion*. Available: www.dansimons.com/videos.html. Last accessed February 2017

Standing, M. (2008) Clinical judgement and decision making in nursing – Nine modes of practice in a revised cognitive continuum. *Journal of Advanced Nursing*, 62(1): 124–34.

Standing, M (2017) *Clinical Judgement and Decision Making for Nursing Students*, 3rd ed. London: Learning Matters (Sage).

Sullivan, E.J. and Decker, P.J. (2003) *Effective Leadership and Management in Nursing*. London: Pearson Prentice Hall.

Syed, M. (2011) *Bounce: The Myth of Talent and the Power of Practice*. New York: Fourth Estate.

Thompson, C. (1999) A conceptual treadmill: the need for 'middle ground' in clinical decision making theory in nursing. *Journal of Advanced Nursing*, 30(5): 1222–9.

Thompson, C. and Dowding, D. (2002). *Decision Making and Judgement in Nursing – An Introduction*. Philadelphia: Churchill Livingstone.

Tversky, A. and Kahneman, D. (1974) Judgment under uncertainty: heuristics and biases. *Science*, 185: 1124–31.

Tversky, A. and Kahneman, D. (1982) Judgments of and by representativeness. In Kahneman, D., Slovic, P. and Tversky, A. (eds), *Judgment Under Uncertainty: Heuristics and Biases*. Cambridge: Cambridge University Press.

UK Sepsis Trust (2016) *Sepsis*. Available: http://sepsistrust.org/. Last accessed February 2017.

Welsh, I. and Lyons, C.M. (2001). Evidence-based care and the case for intuitive and tacit knowledge in clinical assessment and decision making in mental health nursing practice: an empirical contribution to the debate. *Journal of Psychiatric and Mental Health Nursing*, 8: 299–305.

Winters, B.D., Gurses, A.P., Lehmann, H., Sexton, J.B., Rampersad, C.J. and Pronovost, P.J. (2009) Clinical Review Checklist – translating evidence into practice. *Critical Care*, 13(210): 2.

Woollard, M., O'Meara, P. and Munro, G. (2010) What price 90 seconds: is 'Call Connect' a disservice to 999 callers? *Emergency Medical Journal*, 27: 729–30.

World Health Organization (WHO) (2008) *WHO surgical safety checklist and implementation manual*. Available: www.who.int/patientsafety/safesurgery/ss_checklist/en/. Last accessed December 2016.

Yudkowsky, E.S. (2003). *An Intuitive Explanation of Bayes' Theorem*. Available: http://yudkowsky.net/rational/bayes. Last accessed 15th January 2012.

Index